the
body
noble

the
body
noble

20 Minutes to a Hot Body
with Hollywood's Coolest Trainer

derek noble
and
carol colman

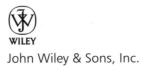

WILEY

John Wiley & Sons, Inc.

Published by John Wiley & Sons, Inc., Hoboken, New Jersey
Published simultaneously in Canada

All photographs by Leslie Whitlock; photographs © Derek Noble

Design and composition by Navta Associates, Inc.

The information contained in this book is not intended to serve as a replacement for professional medical advice. Any use of the information in this book is at the reader's discretion. The author and the publisher specifically disclaim any and all liability arising directly or indirectly from the use or application of any information contained in this book. A health care professional should be consulted regarding your specific situation.

For general information about our other products and services, please contact our Customer Care Department within the United States at (800) 762-2974, outside the United States at (317) 572-3993 or fax (317) 572-4002.

Wiley also publishes its books in a variety of electronic formats. Some content that appears in print may not be available in electronic books. For more information about Wiley products, visit our web site at www.wiley.com.

Library of Congress Cataloging-in-Publication Data:

Noble, Derek, date.
   The body Noble : 20 minutes to a hot body with Hollywood's coolest trainer / Derek Noble.
      p. cm.
   Includes index.
   ISBN-13 978-0-471-72418-1 (cloth)
   ISBN-10 0-471-72418-6 (cloth)
 1. Exercise. 2. Physical fitness. I. Title.
   RA781.N52 2006
   613.7'1—dc22

                                                                    2005022031

Printed in the United States of America

10 9 8 7 6 5 4 3 2 1

In loving memory of my father, The Magnificent Duke Noble,
who guided me with love and wisdom and taught me
that the human body is a temple that must be respected,
strengthened, and maintained.

contents

part three

the body noble lifestyle

acknowledgments

Many thanks to the following people who have been a strong inspirational light in my life as they continue to support my chosen journey:

My friend and coauthor, Carol Colman, who recognized that I had a unique message to relay to the world.

Tom Miller, my editor, and the staff at Wiley who have worked very hard in helping me to create a hip fitness lifestyle book.

My entertainment lawyer, Michael Levine, whose wisdom guides and counsels me in all my business endeavors.

Our agent, Richard Curtis, for his creative input and enthusiasm for this project.

Leslie Whitlock, one of LA's top photographers, whose talent shines through this book; and model Marisa Petroro, a Hollywood actress and model, whose beauty radiates from the inside out.

My mother, Marilyn McGrath, and my two beautiful sisters and their children, who love me unconditionally.

My father, Duke Noble, whose presence I will always feel. He has given me the knowledge and wisdom to dedicate my life to the fitness lifestyle.

My grandmother, Ethel Hayter, who always believed in me and inspired me to always believe in myself. Her support and love provided me with the foundation to focus on my education and career.

My chosen family and friends, Christian Cristiano, Roanna Azar, and Lowell Hall, on whom I can always count to give me the advice and spiritual love that I need.

John Bailey and Muriel Kriss, two friends I can call up any time for good business advice and direction. I also want to thank two special friends for their support—Ron Bush and Mario Solis.

A special thanks to Mariel Kriss for her hard work one Saturday afternoon.

My spiritual teacher, Dr. Reverend Michael Beckwith, of Agape in Los Angeles whose weekly talks have awakened my spirit so that I can continue to use my special gifts to awaken and inspire others.

the body noble method

1

the body noble

How would you like to have a fit, sexy body without ever having to step into a gym? How would you like to reduce stress and feel reenergized? How would you like to be in great shape without ever having to hire a personal trainer, race off to an exercise class, or devote hours of your day to staying fit?

You shouldn't have to turn your life upside down to be fit. You need a fitness program that fits into your schedule—not the other way around. You need a fitness program that works no matter how busy you are and no matter where your day takes you. You need *The Body Noble*.

The Body Noble is based on my innovative training approach, which enables you to maintain a strong, sculpted body in just minutes a day. I began my career as a personal trainer to some of the busiest people on the planet, including high-performance athletes, high-fashion models, and actors who always have to look good. Many of my clients have little or no time to work out, yet I manage to get them into peak condition in record time, without overtaxing their bodies or overstressing their minds. The Body Noble Method can achieve the same fast results for you. It is a safe, simple, fast approach designed to accommodate the busy modern lifestyle.

Some of you may be familiar with my show, *Urban Fitness TV*, the fitness and lifestyle magazine show that airs on FitTV. If you've ever watched *Urban Fitness*, you know that I am on a personal mission to make fitness accessible to everybody. My goal is to dispel the urban myths that discourage many people from even trying to stay fit—such as "You can only get a good workout in a gym," "Staying fit has to disrupt your life," or "Fitness is a luxury that doesn't fit into a fast-paced lifestyle." None of these are true. The Body Noble Method incorporates all the important components of fitness—strength training, stretching, cardio, and relaxation—into one quick, easy-to-follow program that takes about 20 minutes a day. And you can stop paying for that gym membership you never use. You can do a great workout at home in about the same amount of time it would take you to drive to and from the gym. But if you choose to go to a gym, you will find that the Body Noble Method will enable you to work out better and faster there, too.

How is it possible to pack so much into a workout in so little time? When it comes to fitness, quality is far more important than quantity. It doesn't matter whether you do it at home or at a gym, if you work out with the correct technique—which few people actually do—you can achieve spectacular results in a fraction of the time. The reverse is also true: If you don't use the right technique, you can spend hours working out and enjoy few or no results.

a holistic approach

I am passionate that fitness is not about pumping iron or getting bigger muscles. I call myself a fitness lifestyle trainer because I feel that fitness entails living a full, healthy lifestyle, feeling good about your body, and having both the mental and physical energy to achieve your goals. Simply getting someone to go to the gym once or twice a week is not going to make a *long-lasting* change in his or her life, but convincing someone to embrace a fit lifestyle can help facilitate a profound change. The Body Noble Method is as much about enhancing—and enjoying—your life as it is about sculpting and toning your body. It's about eating well, staying centered, and even maintaining the proper posture so that the good results of your workout are not undone by poor muscle alignment. Once you experience true mental and physical well-being, you will not want to go back to your old ways.

The Body Noble Method is also about doing a workout that's right for your body and that doesn't aggravate existing injuries or cause new ones. I studied massage therapy and physical therapy in college, and I draw upon my extensive background in rehabilitation to teach you how to strengthen weak points in your body and protect against injury.

my high-performance life

I come by my interest in fitness naturally. My father, Duke Noble, was a professional wrestler from Alabama who migrated to Toronto in the 1960s. He was one half of the first all–African American tag team. When I was a small boy, I loved it when my dad would bring me to the wrestling ring and hold me up to cheering crowds, which sparked a lifelong interest in performing. As a child, I would spend weekends working out with my dad doing sports, in which I excelled. My dad impressed upon me the need to eat a clean, wholesome diet, and he would often take me to the local health food store, where he would stock up on vitamins and drink freshly squeezed organic juice. Much of the nutrition information he taught me has been incorporated into my own Body Noble Eating Plan, an important component of the Body Noble Method.

I briefly considered a career in medicine, but decided to major in Physical and Health Education at York University in Toronto. To pay my way through college, I worked as an aide in a hospital, where I was assigned to help young paraplegic and quadriplegic patients. Many of my patients were young men in their twenties who were unable to perform the simplest tasks for themselves and who relied on me to do everything for them. Up until then, I had always taken my strong body and good health for granted, and I was profoundly moved by the experience. I came to more fully understand the connection between physical health and mental well-being. Working with these young men taught me an important lesson that I try to pass on to my clients: You are born with one body, and you need to do everything you can to maintain it for a lifetime.

I knew that I enjoyed taking care of people but didn't want to work in a hospital setting. I decided to study sports massage therapy at the Sutherland-Chan Massage Therapy School in Toronto, which would be a great way of incorporating my desire to work with people and my long-standing interest in fitness. The sports massage therapy program was a rigorous undertaking that required more than two thousand classroom hours in the study of anatomy, physiology, rehabilitation, and exercise science. It was the equivalent of a doctorate in muscles, but worth the hard work.

After I completed the training program, I worked as a sports massage therapist at a chiropractic center in Toronto and was appointed head therapist at the Canadian National Tennis Tournament held at York University. One day, John McEnroe walked into the training room complaining of shoulder and hip problems, and I used my blend of massage and stretching therapy to get him back into the game. McEnroe was so impressed with my technique that he offered me a full-time job as his trainer and sports massage therapist. I leapt at the chance to work with the sports icon and to travel with McEnroe and his family during his last year on the ATP tennis circuit.

McEnroe, who was well known for his explosive temper, complained to me that he would sometimes get so angry during a game that he lost his concentration. I suggested that he and I study transcendental meditation as a means to help him better cope with stress. This showed me the importance of incorporating deep breathing and stress reduction into my training regimen.

After a year on the road with McEnroe, I lived in Hollywood, where I was a trainer and sports therapist for celebrities such as Maria Shriver, Michael J. Fox, Tatum O'Neal, and Rutger Hauer. I was lured back to Canada to be a fitness correspondent for CBC, Canada's leading TV network, and I was the host for the International Triathlon series *Very Racy*. I later developed the *Urban Fitness TV* program. I love being on television because I can train thousands of people at a time.

maximize your workout

To get the most out of working out, you need to engage both your mind and your muscles. The Noble Technique explained in this book is one of the unique features of the Body Noble Program. An approach to exercise that allows you to work your muscles more effectively and efficiently than other standard workouts, it consists of three vital components: Touch Training, which I will describe in chapter 5, deep breathing, and visualization. The Noble Technique shows how to isolate each muscle group—and what is more important, how to mentally focus on individual muscles as you work them—so you can get the most out of your workout in the least amount of time.

Once you learn the Body Noble Technique, you're ready to begin the 20-Minute Body Noble Workout, a series of resistance exercises that tones, strengthens, and stretches every important muscle group in your body, from your shoulders to your quads. Ideally, you should do a total body workout at least three times a week.

The stretch component of the Body Noble Workout is as important as the actual workout. If you want to keep your muscles strong and your joints flexible, you have to stretch after working your muscles. Many people, however, have a hit-or-miss attitude about stretching: If they have time at the end of their workout, they do it; if not, they put it off for another day. Pressed for time, many people have eliminated stretching from their exercise routine. Unfortunately, if you don't stretch after weight training, your muscles can become stiff and prone to injury. The major problem is that people don't know how to stretch effectively and efficiently. I show you how to incorporate a quick power stretch into each exercise routine so that every muscle is stretched immediately after working it out.

Cardio, or aerobic training, works your heart and turns up metabolism so you can burn fat and stay lean. You don't need to do a lot of cardio, but you need to do at least 20 minutes every other day. I offer some ingenious ways of adding cardio to your life at your own convenience, in 10-minute intervals, while you're doing other things such as watching television, running an errand, playing with your kids, or shopping.

the world is your gym

With the Body Noble Method, you don't need to invest in a lot of fancy gym equipment for your home. With simple, inexpensive tools such as an exercise ball and an exercise cable, you can do a complete, full-body at-home workout that rivals any gym workout. Once you learn the Body Noble Method, you don't have to be at home to work out. You can tone and strengthen your muscles virtually anywhere, anytime, going about your normal life.

- Stuck at your desk? Stay tight and toned with the Office Pump.
- Sitting in traffic? Put your car in park and do the Traffic Jam Pump for a great upper-body workout.
- Is your plane delayed or are you on a long flight? You can do a full-body Jet Set Fitness Workout.
- It's your turn to clean up the house? Work your upper and lower body with the Dishwashing Upper-Body Pump and the Vacuum-Lunge.
- Glued in front of your TV set? Do the Couch Potato Workout.

The Body Noble Method will show you how to easily and seamlessly incorporate fitness into your life, whether you are having a good week or a bad week.

personalize your workout

Not every workout is for everybody. When I see new clients, I evaluate them to assess which type of workout is best for them and whether they have any specific problems that need to be addressed. To achieve the best results, you need to do a workout that is specific to your body type. There are three basic body types: the lean machine, the muscle maker, and the fat fighter, and each one needs to approach fitness a bit differently. To maintain muscle mass, naturally lean people need to do a more challenging strength-training program (heavier weights and/or more resistance and fewer repetitions) and less cardio. Just the reverse is true for fat fighters: To get lean, they must do more cardio and work with lighter weights and/or resistance and more repetitions to rev up their metabolism. Most people fall into the category of fat fighter—they tend to gain weight easily. Muscle makers are natural athletes who make muscle easily but can get fat quickly if they stop exercising. They need to be vigilant about maintaining a consistent program. To maximize their physical potential, moderately muscular people must do equal amounts of weight training and cardio. How do you know which type you are? I have designed a short questionnaire in chapter 3 to help you identify your strengths and weaknesses so you can personalize your workout.

how to use this book: getting started

I have divided *The Body Noble* into three parts.

part one: the body noble method

The right technique provides a strong foundation for an effective workout. In part one, I teach you everything you need to know about your body so that you can get a great workout each and every time in less time than you ever thought possible. You will learn Touch Training, breathing and visualization exercises, and how to achieve perfect posture. I also give you some important information on how my program can enhance your life and improve your health. I know that some of you may be tempted to skip this section and go right to the Body Noble Workout. Please don't. You will not get optimal results if you don't follow the complete program. You will save yourself a lot of time down the road if you work out correctly in the first place.

part two: the body noble workout

The Body Noble Workout consists of a combination of resistance exercises and stretches that work out every single muscle group using nothing more than an exercise ball and an exercise cable. Once you have mastered the Body Noble Workout, you can move on to the Body Noble On-the-Go Workout, which includes basic exercises that can be done virtually anywhere—at work, commuting to your job, sitting on a park bench, or even washing dishes. The Body Noble Lifestyle Fitness, a variation of the On-the-Go Workout, shows you some fun ways to incorporate basic exercises into your life. And if you get bored with the basic workouts or want to give yourself a real exercise challenge, I offer the Body Noble Challenge, a series of exercises for more advanced people who are progressing rapidly on the program and want to move to another level of fitness.

part three: the body noble lifestyle

Exercise is just one component, albeit an important one, of overall fitness. In part three, I discuss other aspects of staying fit and healthy, including information on nutrition, supplements, how to strengthen your weak links, how to look good, and how to stay motivated.

2

why exercise?

Fitness can improve and extend your life. It can enhance the quality of your life right now and for years to come. You will look better, feel better, and perform better in everything you do.

Stay Slimmer   Weight-loss diets are the wrong way to do it. Dieting typically results in the reduction of weight through the loss of lean body mass and water weight. These changes may prove temporary at best or unhealthy at worst. Exercise, on the other hand, helps you lose the type of weight that causes the most damage to your health and has the biggest impact on your looks: body fat.

Save Your Heart   Exercise helps to keep your arteries from getting blocked with bad stuff called plaque that can cause a heart attack. Exercise is one of the few ways you can raise the level of good cholesterol, which helps the body get rid of bad cholesterol that can clog your arteries and damage your heart. Cardiovascular exercise also helps prevent high blood pressure, a major cause of both heart attack and stroke.

Slow Down the Aging Process   Many people (I'm not one of them) believe that physical decline is an inevitable part of aging. Just tell that to my friend Jack LaLanne, the grandfather of fitness, who at age ninety is still swimming, power walking, and lifting weights every day. Jack was a guest on my show last year, and I can vouch for the fact that he is in better shape than many thirty-year-olds! Much of the physical frailty attributed to aging is actually the result of inactivity. Regular exercise increases life expectancy. The simple truth is, unfit people die younger than fit people, primarily because they fall prey to heart disease, diabetes, and other illnesses that are associated with a sedentary lifestyle, smoking, and poor nutrition.

Reduce the Risk of Cancer   People who do even moderate physical activity are at lower risk of developing several different forms of cancer, including colon cancer in both men and women and breast cancer in women.

Reduce the Risk of Diabetes   The most common form of diabetes, Type 2, develops when the cells of the body become resistant to the hormone insulin, which helps control blood sugar. Insulin resistance occurs when your cells are constantly exposed to high levels of insulin due to a diet that contains too many insulin-producing high-carbohydrate foods (white bread, rolls, chips, snack foods, soda, and other highly processed, refined, sweetened foods). Once rare, Type 2 diabetes is now an epidemic in the United States and the developed world primarily due to the toxic combination of obesity and a sedentary lifestyle. Exercise can reverse the insensitivity to insulin that occurs as a result of being overweight and can lower blood sugar levels. The right diet also plays a significant role in the prevention and treatment of Type 2 diabetes, and my Body Noble Eating Plan is designed to help control blood sugar in a healthy way. If you are already diabetic, you must check with your doctor before changing your diet or embarking on an exercise program.

Save Your Bones   Exercise not only builds stronger muscles, it strengthens your bones and joints. Exercise increases the strength of your tendons and ligaments, the soft tissue that holds your skeleton together. If you have a strong musculoskeletal foundation, you'll be able to pick up those heavy boxes, move the furniture, and rough-house with the kids without risking injury. Exercise also increases flexibility and improves balance and coordination, which makes it much less likely that you will fall and injure yourself as you get older.

Enhance Your Sex Life   Several studies have confirmed that people who exercise have more and better sex than sedentary people. Physical activity works in three primary ways to enhance sexual function. First, it improves cardiovascular fitness, which means that when the time is right, blood can pump freely to the genital region, which is absolutely essential for sexual arousal. Second, exercise boosts the levels of key hormones involved in sexual activity. Third, exercise makes sex better by improving physical stamina, flexibility, and self-esteem.

Improve Your Sleep   Exercise has been proven to be an effective way to treat insomnia and ensure good quality sleep. It tires out your muscles and fatigues your body in a healthy way, allowing you to relax more easily. To get the maximum sleep benefits from exercise, it's important not to exercise too close to bedtime. When you work out, your body temperature rises and you secrete adrenaline, a stimulant. It takes about two to three hours for your body to return to normal, so try to exercise at least three hours before you go to bed so that you're not too pumped to sleep.

Get Happy   Studies demonstrate that a regular exercise program can often be just as effective as medication or psychotherapy in treating symptoms of depression. Exercise also relieves stress, one of the most harmful side effects of modern life. Stress makes you anxious, irritable, and depressed. Chronic stress can cause an increase in blood pressure, which is bad for your heart. After you've done the Body Noble Program for a week or two, you'll see how good you feel.

Stay Smarter   Moderate levels of exercise can improve performance on memory and thinking tasks. In other words, it makes you smarter. Regular physical activity also increases concentration and the ability to multitask, and it appears to enhance creativity. Physical activity increases blood flow to the brain, which gives your brain more nourishment and makes you feel instantly alert.

I've given you some great reasons to follow the Body Noble Program. You now have both the skills and the motivation you need to get the most out of the program. You are now ready to begin the Body Noble Workout.

3

which body noble
are you?

To get the best results from the Body Noble Program, you need to do a workout that is specifically designed for your body type. As I've said, there are three basic body types: the lean machine, the muscle maker, and the fat fighter, and each type needs to approach fitness a bit differently. To make and maintain muscle mass, lean machines need a challenging strength-training program that employs heavier weights or more resistance and fewer repetitions, and a less challenging cardio program. Conversely, fat fighters need a challenging cardio program coupled with a moderate strength-training program that employs lighter weights and/or resistance and more repetitions of each exercise. Muscle makers, natural athletes who make muscle easily but can become fat quickly if they stop exercising, must do equally challenging weight training and cardio programs. They need to be vigilant about maintaining a consistent program. Most of us fall into the category of fat fighter. We tend to gain weight easily, and we need to incorporate more aerobic exercises—what I call cardio breaks—into our routines, and do more repetitions of each exercise with lower weights to rev up our metabolism.

When I meet new clients, I evaluate them to determine the type of workout that best suits them and whether they have any specific problems that need to be addressed. Then I help them tailor their workouts to get the best results. I'd love to work with each of you individually, but since I can't, I will do the next best thing. I have designed a short questionnaire to help you identify your body type so that you can follow the Noble Method that best suits your needs. By the time you have finished answering these few questions, you will know which body type best correlates with your own. Throughout the book, I will address the needs of the three specific body types so that you can get the most out of your workout. Keep in mind that there is no good or bad body type. For the purposes of this book, please be honest and answer the questions based on who you are now, not who you once were or who you aspire to be. With the proper program, any body type can achieve terrific results and look great.

An effective workout is also a safe workout! I don't want you doing things that could hurt your body or aggravate an existing injury. Please review chapter 14, Strengthening Your Weak Links, to see how you can further modify your workout to accommodate any weakness or injury.

Your Shape

What shape best describes your body?

1. Lean and angular _____
2. Broader on top and narrower on bottom (inverted triangle) _____
3. Round (apple- or pear-shaped) _____

Lean Machine: Is This You?

Check yes or no for each of the four statements below.

1. No matter how much I eat, I can't seem to keep the weight on regardless of my activity level.   Yes _____ No _____
2. I worry that I look too bony.   Yes _____ No _____
3. I can't find any fat on my body, not even in places where I'd like to see some, such as on my rear end.   Yes _____ No _____
4. I look like a ballet dancer or a marathon runner.
   Yes _____ No _____

Muscle Maker: Is This You?

Check yes or no for each of the four statements below.

1. When I don't work out regularly, my muscles turn to flab. Yes _____ No _____

2. When I'm in shape, my shoulders and chest are bigger than my waist and hips. Yes _____ No _____

3. When I'm working out, I can eat all I want without getting fat, but when I stop working out and eat all I want, I get fat very quickly. Yes _____ No _____

4. When I start working out—even if I haven't worked out for a long time—I get well toned very quickly, within a few weeks. Yes _____ No _____

Fat Fighter: Is This You?

Check yes or no for each of the four statements below.

1. I can pinch more than an inch of fat on my body. Yes _____ No _____

2. If I don't carefully watch what I eat, I put on weight very easily. Yes _____ No _____

3. Weight tends to concentrate around my waist and hips. Yes _____ No _____

4. When I start working out, it can take up to several months before I see any significant results. Yes _____ No _____

understanding your score

Your Shape

- If you checked off *lean and angular*, you are probably a lean machine, but you will know more when you finish reading these pages.

- If you checked off *broader on top and narrower on bottom*, you are probably a muscle maker, but you will know more when you finish reading these pages.

- If you checked off *round*, you are probably a fat fighter, but you will know more when you finish reading these pages.

Lean Machine: Is This You?

If you answered yes to three out of four questions, you are a *lean machine*. Please read more about lean machines beginning at the bottom of this page.

Muscle Maker: Is This You?

If you answered yes to three out of four questions, you are a *muscle maker*. Please read more about muscle makers on page 19.

Fat Fighter: Is This You?

If you answered yes to three out of four questions, you are a *fat fighter*. Please read more about fat fighters on page 21.

By now, most of you will know your body type, but a rare few may not be sure. Let the first question be the tie breaker. If you are debating between two types, take a hard look at yourself in the mirror. Are you lean and angular like a lean machine? Are you broader on top and narrower on the bottom like a muscle maker? Are you round like a fat fighter? Let your reflection in the mirror be your guide.

can your body type change?

Yes! As we age, our metabolism slows down. At the same time, many of us become less active. As a result, a young lean machine or muscle maker can become a middle-aged fat fighter.

lean machine

Your friends are jealous that you can eat up a storm and never gain an ounce, but you are self-conscious about looking too scrawny. When you look in the mirror, all you see are the bones jutting out from under your skin. You desperately want a more shapely, well-toned body. The good news is, once you put some muscle on those bones, you're going to look fantastic!

Fortunately, with the right kind of workout your lean machine body will make muscle very quickly. The key to success is to do resistance training at high enough levels to stimulate muscle growth. Since you don't have much fat to burn off, your muscles will respond quickly to a high-intensity workout. Within a matter of weeks, you will see your body go from too skinny to shapely and strong. The biggest mistake lean machines make is doing too much cardio, which will actually promote the destruction of muscle, and not working muscles hard enough to get significant results.

Workout Tips   The fastest way for lean machines to grow muscle is to do fewer repetitions per set (around 8 to 10) at a high-intensity level. After your initial warm up set, you should work at an intensity level of 4 or 5 on the Body Noble Rating Scale (see chapter 4), which shows you a simple way to determine how hard you are working. Don't overdo the cardio. Three cardio breaks a week is enough to keep your heart strong without tearing down your muscle.

Diet Tips   Men should eat between 2,000 and 3,500 calories a day, and women between 1,200 and 1,500 calories a day just to maintain their weight. I don't want you to actually count calories, but do eat three *full* meals plus snacks!

muscle maker

Muscle makers have a natural tendency to make muscle. Muscle makers tend to be natural athletes—they're the high school jocks who excel at sports or even real pros. They're lucky—up to a point. When muscle makers are physically active, they have a well-toned, nicely sculpted physique. But keeping that great body takes work. Unfortunately, once muscle makers hit their twenties and thirties, and find themselves sitting behind a desk all day or taking care of kids, they often stop getting regular exercise. So all their wonderful muscle turns to flab. Muscle is the most metabolically active tissue in the body (it burns a lot more calories than fat). Exercise stimulates muscles to keep burning fat. When you stop exercising, however, all that muscle turns into sluggish fat and doesn't burn calories anymore, it just makes more fat cells.

If you're a muscle maker, work at maintaining your muscle or you will lose it. Resistance training is extremely important to restore strength and vitality to sagging muscles and to prevent existing muscle from turning into fat. You also need to incorporate equal amounts of cardio into your workout to burn off any excess fat and turn up your metabolism so you keep burning fat.

Workout Tips Your goal is to rescue your body from the layer of fat that is hiding your muscles. With a little effort, you can have a firmer, better-toned body. You will need to maintain muscle if you already have it or restore the muscle that you may have lost over time. Since it's easy for you to make muscle, your goal is to work at a medium-to-hard intensity level (around 4) on the Body Noble Rating Scale (see chapter 4), which shows you a simple way to determine how hard you are working. Do 10 to 15 reps per set and don't neglect your cardio! You should do 3 to 5 cardio breaks a week to periodically stoke your metabolism to keep burning fat.

Diet Tips Muscle makers can typically eat generous amounts of food when they're working out and must pare down when they're not. It may take some trial and error to figure out exactly how much you can eat and still maintain your ideal body. If you haven't been exercising in a while, you will find that an increase in activity will give your metabolism a much needed boost, and you may be able to eat more and keep the weight off. A word of caution: If you stop working out, you will lose your muscle, and have to cut back on calories.

fat fighter

Do you feel that you are on a perpetual diet? Is it getting harder and harder to keep the weight off? Does fat seem to congregate around your waist or hips? You are a fat fighter—your body has a natural tendency to make fat and store fat, not burn fat. If you're not careful about eating carefully and working out, you will get fat and flabby very quickly. You can have a trim, well-toned, attractive body once you incorporate the right strategy. A resistance training program will help develop metabolically active muscle so that you begin burning off fat more efficiently. You must also be vigilant about doing your cardio—every day if possible—if you need to lose weight. Cardio stimulates fat burning.

Your ideal body may not be a model size two or even a size eight for a woman, or a perfect thirty-four waist for a man. It doesn't matter! Your goal is to lean down your body so that it is well defined, healthy, and looking good. Remember, it's all about feeling sexy and comfortable in your own skin, not about measuring up to some impossible standard. With a little work, a fit fat fighter can have a really hot body.

Workout Tips Before you can start making muscle, you need to burn off the fat. Cardio is an extremely important part of your workout routine. You should strive to do 4 to 5 cardio breaks a week. Do your resistance training at a moderate to hard intensity level (around 3 to 4) on the Body Noble Rating Scale (see chapter 4), which shows you how to determine how hard you are working. You have to do more repetitions than the lean machine or the muscle maker—15 to 20 repetitions per set is ideal. The moderate intensity, high-repetition workout will turn up your metabolism and promote fat burning.

Diet Tips Fat fighters can put on excess pounds very easily if they are not careful about what they eat. Be vigilant about watching your portion sizes so that you don't routinely take in excess calories. Avoid high-calorie, high-sugar, or high-fat junk food such as soda, candy bars, or chips. Snacking on bad stuff can be your downfall because it's much harder for you to burn off excess calories. In particular, fat fighters have to limit their consumption of high-sugar carbohydrates (basically all unprocessed white flour products including white bread and pasta), which are readily stored in the body as fat. At the same time, restrict your intake of saturated fat (found in meat and full-fat dairy products) because it is the hardest fat for your body to burn.

Lean Machine Workout Tips

Do two sets of every exercise, 8 to 10 repetitions per set.
Work out at an intensity level of 4 to 5 on the Body Noble Rating Scale.
Do 3 cardio breaks a week.

Muscle Maker Workout Tips

Do two sets of every exercise, 10 to 15 reps per set.
Work out at an intensity level of around 4 on the Body Noble Rating Scale.
Do 3 to 5 cardio breaks a week.

Fat Fighter Workout Tips

Do two sets of every exercise, 15 to 20 repetitions.
Work out at a moderate to hard intensity level (around 3 to 4) on the Body Noble Rating Scale.
Do 4 to 5 cardio breaks a week.

4

noble resistance: putting the work back into your workout

The goal of a good workout is to burn fat and make muscle. If you don't work out with the right level of intensity (that is, if you don't work your muscle hard enough), you're wasting your time.

When you work a muscle harder than usual, you make the working muscle hypertrophy, or get bigger. When you pick up a weight that is heavier than anything you normally lift in daily life or when you use your own body weight to create resistance (as you do if you are doing situps correctly), your muscle fibers rub against each other, causing small, microscopic tears. In the short run, you are injuring your muscle fibers, but in the end, it's for a good cause. The muscle responds to the injury by growing new muscle cells, which ultimately makes it bigger and stronger. Women, take note: I've had many female clients say to me, "Derek, I don't want big muscles, so why should I work out!" Muscle tissue is very compact compared to fat. When you burn off fat and make muscle, your body looks slimmer but well sculpted. Muscle cells are also much more metabolically active than fat cells, which means that muscle cells burn more calories, making you trimmer. I know that many body builders have huge muscles and look very big, but they follow a completely different style of working out and eating than what I recommend in the Body Noble Program. In addition, I'm sad to say, many pros (or wannabe pros) take steroids and other performance-enhancement drugs to speed things along. Most of us don't have to worry about getting too big from working out. Women simply don't make enough male hormones to create huge muscles—and neither do most men.

think negative

To get the best results from your workout, you need to work out correctly. Every motion in an exercise is important to building muscle—from start to finish. Unfortunately, many people concentrate on the first part of an exercise, the concentric contraction or positive motion, but neglect the second part, the eccentric or negative motion, which is even more important in creating muscle. For example, when you do a bicep curl in the positive motion, you squeeze your bicep (your upper arm muscle) as you lift the weight close to your chest. In the second part of the exercise, the negative motion, you release the weight to the starting position. You should be working equally hard when you release the weight as when you first lifted it. People often get careless when they release the weight, and let momentum take over. This is a mistake because you actually use more muscle fibers when you have to move the weight against momentum than you do when you lift it up. If you don't work at releasing the weight slowly, carefully, and with absolute control, you are cheating yourself out of the full benefit of your workout. That's why I tell my clients to count "1, 2" on the positive motion, and to count "1, 2, 3, 4" on the negative motion for every exercise. The longer count on the negative motion forces you to slow down and not rush through the exercise when the going gets tough.

To make the most of the precious time you spend working out, work at the right level of intensity for your body type. For example, to gain mass, lean machines should do resistance training at the highest level of intensity that they can. On the other hand, fat fighters can't work at an intensity that burns them out too quickly, because they need to have energy left for those extra fat-burning reps. Muscle makers need to find a happy medium that gives them a meaningful workout but doesn't underwork or overwork their muscles.

How do you know which level of intensity is right for you? At first it may seem a bit confusing to hear advice like "Strive to work at the highest level of intensity that you can," or " I want you to work at just below your maximum level." Until you actually begin to follow the exercise program, you may not quite understand what this is all about. But I promise, once you get going, it will seem obvious.

To make it easy to figure out the right level of intensity for you, I have designed the Body Noble Rating Scale based on a rating of 1 to 5. In the beginning, you may need to refer to it often to help you reach your optimal level of intensity. Within a short time, though, it will become second nature, and you will think to yourself, "I'm working at a Level 3," or "It's time to switch to Level 5."

Body Noble Rating Scale

Level 1: This is a nice light workout. It feels good, and I can keep going.

Level 2: I'm starting to feel my muscles burn.

Level 3: I can really feel my muscles working hard, but I still have more to give.

Level 4: It's getting a lot tougher . . . but I can still do most of my reps if I really try.

Level 5: Wow! I'm maxing out fast. . . . I can't do much more.

When you first begin working out, use the Body Noble Rating Scale as a gauge to help you figure out what your workout should feel like. Within a short time, you will know the difference between a light Level 2 warm-up and a I'm-giving-all-I-got Level 5. Periodically, you may need to refer back to the Body Noble Rating Scale to make sure that you are getting the most out of your workout. If things are beginning to get too easy for you or you feel that you've stopped making progress, you're ready to take it up a notch and work harder. As you get stronger, what once felt like Level 3 or 4 may now be your new Level 2 or 3. Don't get complacent. To maintain a sexy, fit Body Noble, you will need to stay on top of your workout so you can stay on top of your game.

5

the body noble technique

The Body Noble Technique teaches you how to best prepare your body and mind for a successful workout. The Noble Technique is the reason the Body Noble Method is so effective and is why my clients are able to achieve twice the results in half the time. Some trainers require people to do 3 or even 4 sets of a particular exercise. What a waste of time! On the Body Noble Program, you only need to do 2 sets of any one exercise because you will do it so effectively, you don't need to do more. That's why you're able to do a full-body workout in about 20 minutes.

There are three components to the Body Noble Technique: Touch Training, deep breathing, and visualization. The Noble Technique is not just for beginners. Before every workout session, I devote 2 to 3 minutes to reviewing the Noble Technique so that every workout is a great workout. Once you learn the fundamentals of the Noble Technique, you will be able to run through them quickly—but you have to learn them first. Once you do, you will *feel* the difference in your workout, and you will *see* the difference in your body.

I believe that you need to understand how your body works before you work out. You wouldn't get in a car and start driving without knowing the rules of the road, and you shouldn't start an exercise program without knowing how to work your body safely and effectively. Do you know which muscles are which, and what they do? Please review the Muscle Map below. It will help you identify your muscles and give you a better understanding of where they are and what they do.

body noble muscle map

Front View

1. CHEST MUSCLES (*Pectorals Major and Minor*)
Pecs help you push things away from your body. You use them when you mow the lawn, vacuum, or push a shopping cart or baby stroller.

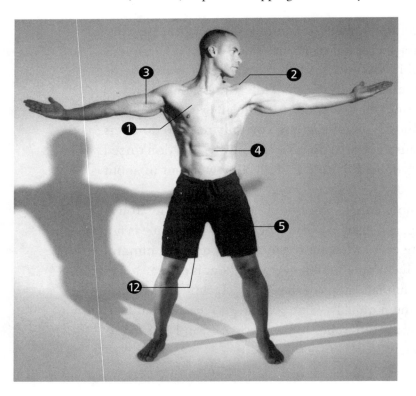

2. SHOULDER MUSCLES (*Deltoids*)
These muscles help you raise objects above your head. You use them when you put a suitcase in the overhead storage compartment of an airplane, or put dishes away in a kitchen cabinet. (That's why so many people come home from vacations with sore shoulder muscles!)

3. FRONT UPPER-ARM MUSCLES (*Biceps*)
These muscles help you carry things. You use them when you haul a bag of groceries home from the supermarket or hold a baby.

4. ABDOMINAL MUSCLES (*"Abs"*)

These muscles are part of the mid-core area of your body that keeps you upright and in good posture. You use them every time you sit, stand, lift, or move.

5. FRONT LEG MUSCLES (*Quadriceps*)

These muscles are essential for walking, climbing, and bending down. You need strong leg muscles to walk up steps or bend down to pick things up.

Back View

6. WIDE BACK MUSCLES AND (6A) UPPER-BACK MUSCLES (*Trapezius, Latismus*) AND NECK MUSCLES

These muscles keep your head upright. You use them when you're working at your computer or driving a car.

7. MID-BACK MUSCLES (*Rhomboids, Teres Major and Minor*)

These muscles help you when you pull things toward you. You use them when you work out on a rowing machine, drag a vacuum back and forth, or bring your fork to your mouth.

8. REAR UPPER-ARM MUSCLES (*Triceps*)

These muscles help you when you push your body up from a sitting position. You use your upper arm muscles when you lift yourself out of a chair or bench or off your exercise mat.

9. LOWER-BACK MUSCLES (*Erector Spinae*)

These important muscles stabilize your back so you don't fall over. You use them when you bend over from the waist to lift things.

10. BUTT MUSCLES (*Gluteal*)

Glutes are powerful muscles that allow you to propel yourself forward without falling. You use them to walk and run.

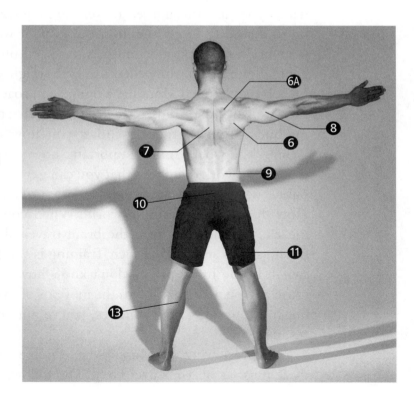

11. REAR LEG MUSCLES *(Hamstrings)*
These muscles support the thighs and butt. If they are tight, you run the risk of lower-back injuries. You use them to walk and climb steps.

12. INNER THIGHS *(Hip Adductors)* **AND OUTER THIGHS** *(Hip Abductors)*
These muscles are important for hip and back stability. You use them every time you pivot or step to the side. Sports that involve lateral movements, such as tennis, volleyball, basketball, and football, utilize these muscles.

13. CALF MUSCLES *(Gastrocnemius)*
These muscles provide stability to the lower part of your body. You use them to stand up tall on the tips of your toes.

get in touch with your muscles

Effective strength training is not a mindless, mechanical activity in which you rush through each exercise as quickly as possible and move on to the next. To get the most out of your workout, you need to use your brain to work your muscles. As I tell my clients, "No brain, no gain!" Before I allow my clients to lift a weight or use an exercise cable, I teach them Touch Training, a unique approach to exercise that allows them to work their muscles more effectively and efficiently than other methods. Touch Training shows you how to isolate each muscle group—and what is more important, how to visualize individual muscles as you work them—so that you can get the most out of your workout in the least amount of time. You want to feel your muscles working. How does Touch Training work? When you think about working a muscle, the message from the brain travels down to the muscle, and the muscle is activated. Touch Training is similar to turning on a light switch in the brain: If you don't know how to properly activate your muscles, you may go through the motions of working out, but if you are not fully engaging your muscles, you're not going to achieve the best results.

After reviewing the Muscle Map, I'd like you to identify and isolate these muscles on your own body. The following Touch Training exercises will help make you aware of how it feels to contract and squeeze each of your individual muscle groups. This is excellent preparation for the Body Noble Workout. When you begin working out, it is essential that you know how to isolate your individual muscles so that you get the full benefit of my program. I recommend that you do each of these exercises at least twice before starting the Body Noble Workout. Please review the Touch Training system periodically to make sure that you are using your muscles correctly.

touch training

Upper Portion of the Abdominal Muscles *("Abs")*

1. Stand in a comfortable position with your legs shoulder width apart, your back straight, and your head facing forward.

2. Place both hands right above your abs.

3. With four fingers from each hand, gently massage your abs in a circular, forward motion. Breathe in and out. As you massage the area, squeeze and contract your abs. Exhale and hold the contraction for 5 seconds before releasing it. Feel the squeeze.

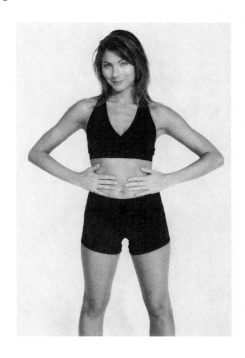

4. Keep massaging your abs, and feel them go in and out with each contraction.

5. Close your eyes and visualize your abs. See the squeeze. See your abs go in and out as you keep squeezing. Say to yourself, *I can feel my abs working now. I can feel my abs relaxing now.*

Every time you work your abs, remember what this looks like and feels like.

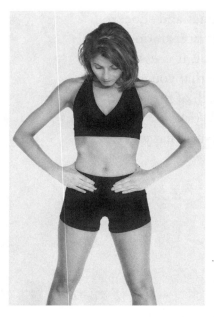

Lower Portion of the Abdominal Muscles
("Abs" Interior and Exterior Obliques)

1. Stand in a comfortable position with your legs shoulder width apart, your back straight, and your head down toward your chin, looking at your abdomen.

2. Breathe in and out. Press and feel below your abs using four fingers and visualize the muscles working as you contract and release your abs, in and out.

3. Imagine that a small water balloon is inside your lower abs. As you exhale, try to squeeze as much water out of the balloon as possible. Keep squeezing until you wring out every last drop of water. Feel the squeeze deep within your muscles.

Chest Muscles *(Pectoralis Major and Minor)*

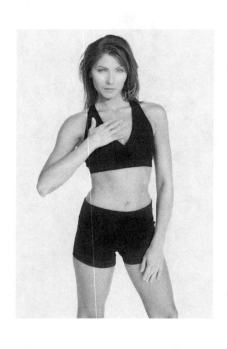

1. Stand in a comfortable position with your legs shoulder width apart, your back straight, and your head facing forward.

2. Bend your right elbow 90 degrees and place your right arm in front of you.

3. Place your hand on your right chest muscle. Squeeze in your chest as you roll your left arm in toward your body.

4. Exhale and hold the squeeze for 5 seconds. Feel the chest squeeze. Close your eyes and see your chest muscle expanding and contracting. Say to yourself, *I can feel my chest muscle working hard. When I work my chest, this is the muscle I need to work.*

5. Repeat with your left arm, touching your left chest muscle.

Front Upper-Arm Muscles *(Biceps)*

1. Standing up, drop your arms straight by your sides. With your right hand grab your left upper arm, or bicep.

2. Squeeze your left arm with your right hand as you contract your left bicep muscle, then release it. Feel your left bicep expand and contract. Exhale and hold the bicep squeeze for 5 seconds. Close your eyes. See the squeeze and feel your bicep expand and contract. Think to yourself, *This is how my bicep feels when I'm working it.*

3. Repeat with your left hand and right bicep.

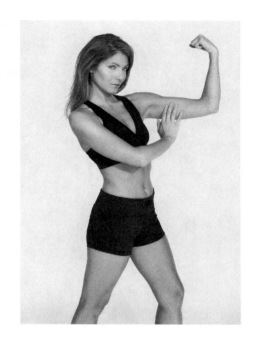

Rear Upper-Arm Muscles *(Triceps)*

1. Standing up, drop your arms straight by your sides. Put your right hand on the side of your left upper arm, the tricep.

2. Squeeze your right arm as you contract your left tricep muscle. Feel your left tricep expand and contract. Exhale and hold the tricep squeeze for 5 seconds. Close your eyes. See the squeeze. See your tricep expand and contract. Remember how your tricep feels when you are working it.

3. Repeat with your left hand and right tricep.

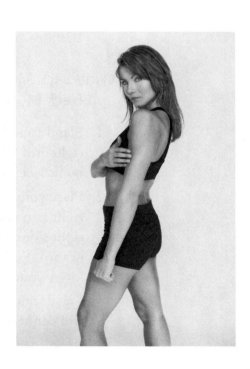

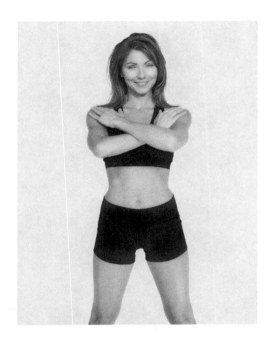

Shoulder Muscles *(Deltoids)*

1. Stand up straight with your feet shoulder width apart. Cross your arms in front of your chest and place each hand on the front of the opposite shoulder.

2. Tense the round muscles on top of your shoulders. Feel them go in and out. Do the right shoulder, do the left shoulder, and then do both shoulders together.

3. Repeat the exercise.

Wide Back Muscles *(Trapezius, Latisimus)* and Neck Muscles

1. Stand straight with your feet shoulder width apart. Bend your right arm 90 degrees and extend out from the side of your body. Keep your hand straight in the air.

2. Place your left hand on your side back muscles. Lower your right arm and elbow closer to your body and contract the right side of your back muscles as you lower your arm inward. Feel your right side lat muscles squeezing as you lower your arm down and in.

3. Exhale and hold the squeeze for 5 seconds. Close your eyes and connect to this large muscle group.

4. Repeat with your left arm and right back muscle.

Mid-Back Muscles *(Rhomboids, Teres Major and Minor)*

1. Stand straight with your back and shoulders against a wall.
2. Squeeze your back muscles (in the middle) as you press your back into the wall. Feel the squeeze in your back as you tighten your back muscles.
3. Exhale while holding the squeeze for 5 seconds. Close your eyes. Visualize your back muscles contracting as you work them.

Lower-Back Muscles *(Erector Spinae)*

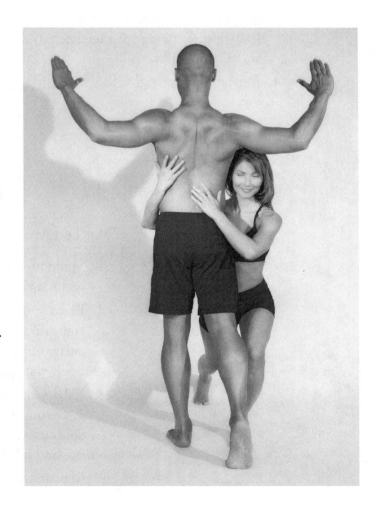

1. Stand straight with your arms bent at 90 degrees and extended out to the side for balance.
2. Extend your right leg backward as you contract your lower back and buttock muscles. Feel the squeeze in your lower back.
3. Exhale and hold the squeeze for 5 seconds with each leg. Close your eyes and visualize your back muscles contracting as you work them.
4. Go back to the starting position and reverse, doing the exercise on your left leg.

Front Leg Muscles *(Quadriceps)*

1. Stand up straight with your feet shoulder width apart.

2. Place your left hand on your left thigh muscle. Extend your knee straight out in front of you. As you extend your knee, feel your thigh muscles contract.

3. Exhale and hold the contraction for 5 seconds. Close your eyes. See your thigh muscle tightening. Feel how hard it's working. Bring your leg back to the starting position.

4. Repeat on your right side.

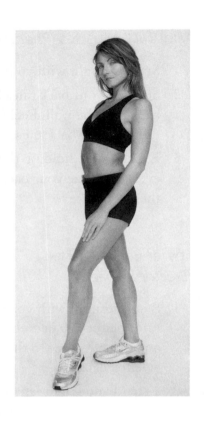

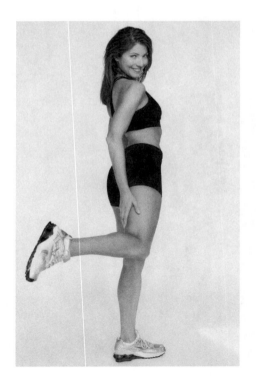

Rear Leg Muscles *(Hamstrings)*

1. Stand up straight with your feet shoulder width apart.

2. Place your right hand on the back of your right thigh muscle. Flex your knee and curl your leg in toward your butt muscles. Feel your quad muscles contract.

3. Exhale and hold the hamstring squeeze for 5 seconds. Close your eyes and see the contraction. Bring your leg back to the starting position.

4. Repeat on your left side.

Butt Muscles
(Gluteal, or "Glutes")

1. Stand up tall with your feet shoulder width apart. Place both hands on your glute muscles under your butt.

2. Press down into your feet as you thrust your pelvis up toward the ceiling. Feel the squeeze in your butt as you move up. Exhale and hold the squeeze for 5 seconds. Relax.

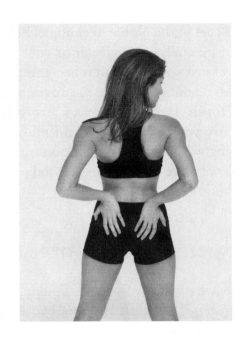

Calf Muscles *(Gastrocnemius)*

1. Stand up straight with your feet shoulder width apart.

2. Move your left leg behind you. Reach for your left calf muscle with your left hand. Press your left toes into the ground as you raise yourself up on the tips of your toes.

3. Exhale and hold the squeeze for 5 seconds. Feel the contraction as you squeeze your left calf muscle. Feel the shape and form of the muscle with your hand. Relax. Repeat the exercise with your right leg.

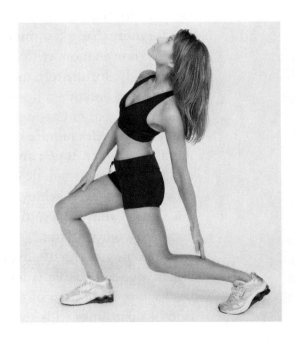

As part of the Noble Technique, before you begin each workout, you should mentally review each of your Touch Training exercises. When you feel that your workout is becoming stale or that you're not getting all you should out of your fitness program, it's a sign you may need to review your Touch Training exercises. Are you squeezing your muscles properly? Are you working the right muscle for each exercise? Your Touch Training will help get you back on track.

Now you're ready for the second part of your Noble Technique, deep breathing.

body noble deep-breathing exercises

I know what many of you are thinking: *I don't need breathing lessons, I've been breathing my whole life!* You'd be shocked to learn that you're probably doing it all wrong.

The purpose of breathing is to bring oxygen into your blood so it can be distributed throughout the cells and tissues of your body. Oxygen is essential for the production of energy by our cells, which is why we can't live for more than a few minutes without taking a breath. Think about it: Oxygen is even more critical for our immediate survival than either food or water. Unfortunately, most people do not breathe correctly or effectively. They breathe in just enough air to keep their heart pumping and brain going, but not enough to maximize performance. When you work out, your muscles require extra blood and oxygen so they can grow bigger and stronger. If you are a shallow breather, as most people are, you are depriving your muscle cells of the oxygen boost that could make the difference between achieving your fitness potential or falling short of your goals. You will also find that you run out of steam before you can complete your workout.

Breathing correctly involves fully engaging the diaphragm muscle under your ribs so that you fill your lungs with air. Your lungs extend all the way to the bottom of your rib cage. Most people fill the upper portion of their lungs with air, but fail to breathe deeply enough to inflate the bottom portion. You must breathe in and out through your nose in order to fill your lungs to their full capacity. Mouth breathing is not as effective, and will tire you out faster.

Deep breathing has proven health benefits. Numerous scientific studies show that deep breathing exercises can lower your blood pressure, relieve hot flashes in menopausal women, reduce stress, and improve your athletic performance. As anyone who has ever practiced yoga breathing exercises knows, deep breathing is a great stress reliever.

Eager to get started? The simple deep-breathing exercises described below will help retrain you to breathe properly. As your body becomes more energized with oxygen, you will immediately feel a positive difference in terms of mood and stamina. I recommend doing a few minutes of deep-breathing exercises before you work out. You will feel calmer, more focused, and more alert.

Take a Noble Breath

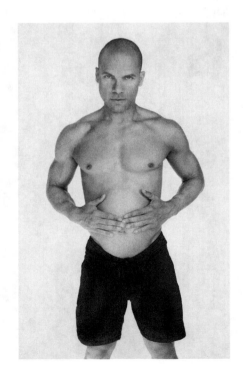

1. Stand in a comfortable position with your feet shoulder width apart. Close your eyes and relax for a few seconds.

2. Breathe in deeply through your nose. Distend your belly up while you are inhaling so your belly fills up with air. Look down and watch your belly rise.

3. When you have filled your belly with as much air as you can take in, stop and hold your breath. Try to hold it for about 10 seconds.

4. Put your hands on your diaphragm muscle, which lies right under your rib cage. Put your hands into the muscle as you exhale your breath. You will feel your diaphragm muscle pushing up under your rib cage. Exhale for 10 more seconds.

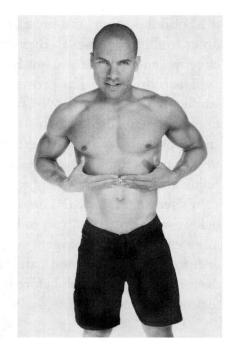

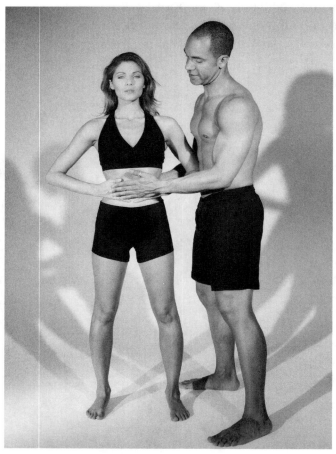

Did you feel your lungs stretching out? Did you feel your diaphragm muscles working hard? Good. Keep practicing for 5 more minutes. Now sit up in a chair and do the same exercise. Concentrate on inflating your belly. Memorize how you feel when you breathe in deeply, your belly expands, and your diaphragm pushes in. Feel the rhythm of deep breathing. Keep practicing for another 5 minutes.

How do you feel? This exercise probably feels both good

and bad to you at the same time—your body loves the extra oxygen, but you're working overtime to breathe it in. By now you have a sense of how to breathe deeply. After a few minutes of deep breathing, you undoubtedly feel relaxed and refreshed. But if you don't keep practicing, you will quickly fall back to your bad habits. Take a day or two to practice this technique. Keep at it. I promise that the more you practice, the easier it will become, and soon you will be breathing deeply and correctly without giving it a thought.

Breathing is fundamental to fitness. Oxygen is as important a fuel for your body as food is, only oxygen is calorie-free. You can breathe as deeply as you want and not gain weight. Moreover, the extra oxygen actually speeds up chemical reactions in your body that help burn off the calories from food faster. So keep practicing your deep breathing—your body will love you for it.

visualization: seeing is believing

The expression "Seeing is believing" takes on a special meaning when it comes to fitness. If you want to *achieve it*, you must first *see it*. When you work a muscle, it is critical that you actually see the muscle in your mind's eye. Before you pick up a weight or pull an exercise cable, you must say to yourself, *What muscle am I working?* In Touch Training, you learned how to physically isolate your muscles. Now I want you to learn how to create a mental image of each muscle—to visualize the muscle in your brain. I want you to visualize the working muscle each time you squeeze and release it. How does visualization improve your workout? When you exercise a muscle, the actual process begins in the brain, not the body. In a fraction of a second, your brain sends a message down through your nervous system, telling the cells in your muscles they are being summoned into action. When your brain is truly focused on the muscle that you are working, you not only engage more muscle cells, you work them more effectively. You get faster and better results. I can actually see it happen when I'm training someone. I can see a real difference in their workout when they are making that mental connection and their muscles are really firing.

Over time, seeing the muscles you are working will become second nature. Each time you begin an exercise, automatically say to yourself, *I know what muscle I'm working*, and you will know how to visually stimulate your muscle to get the most out of your workout. Many people go to the gym a lot, but they really don't know what muscle groups they're working and what fibers are being isolated. They don't get a good result. I practice what I preach, and it shows. I train 2 to 3 times a week, but my body looks like I train 6 days a week. Visualization helps me maximize my results without overworking my body, and it will work for you, too.

see your body noble

I believe that it's important to have a fitness goal, a vision of the *perfect body for you*. I call it your Body Noble. I use the word "perfect" advisedly. I urge clients to look in magazines and cut out pictures of people with similar body types whom they aspire to look like. The key is to have a realistic picture of your ideal body. If you are a lean machine male, you are never going to look like a massive body builder, but you can still have a strong, well-defined body. If you are a female fat fighter, you're never going to look like a size-two fashion model, but you can still be trim, shapely, and not flabby. Have an image in your head of your Body Noble, and use that image to motivate you to stick to the program. Think of your Body Noble when you need an incentive to do your workout or skip a fattening dessert. When you actually achieve your Body Noble, use your inner vision of your ideal body as an inspiration to keep going.

visualization exercise

Before you begin your exercise routine, take a moment to sit quietly and focus on your body. Begin with your deep-breathing exercises. Breathe deeply in and out. Then use your brain to connect to your muscles. Visualize your Body Noble. See yourself in your perfect body. Once you have an overall picture of your Body Noble, you can begin to isolate certain areas of your body. Think about how good specific parts of your body can look—your neck, your chest, your arms, your shoulders, your abs, your back, your butt, your legs. Now go back and think about your entire body. Restore that image of your Body Noble.

In the next chapter, I'll show you how to achieve perfect posture.

6

body noble posture: stand, sit, and sleep right

Every time I work out with a client, I begin each session with a posture check to make sure his or her body is in proper alignment. Why do I spend precious minutes on posture? As I tell my clients, trying to start a fitness program with poor posture is like trying to build a new home on shaky ground. If you don't build your house on a solid foundation, it will eventually crumble, and the same is true for your body. If you try to build a core conditioning program on a poorly supported foundation, you will very likely develop muscle imbalances that will ultimately lead to injury.

Posture is the missing link in fitness. It doesn't get the attention it deserves, and as a result, people are getting hurt. Look around any gym and you will see that many of the people doing cardio are hunched over treadmills and stair-step machines with their shoulders tense and rotated forward. What's wrong with this picture? The slouched, forward position of the shoulders throws the body out of alignment, placing undue pressure on the shoulders, neck, back, and knees. If you exercise for too long in this position, you can throw your back out or develop neck and shoulder problems. Pretty soon, you won't be able to exercise at all. It's not just the people doing cardio who are at risk. Move on to the weight room and you will see people lifting heavy weights with their knees locked in a stiff position, which places excess strain on their back. This poor posture not only hurts their knees, it can also do serious harm to their back.

It's just as important to maintain good posture when you're going about your everyday life. When you stand in line at the bank or at the checkout counter in a store, if you round your shoulders and stiffen your knees, you are at risk of straining your back. If you sit slumped over a computer screen all day, you are placing undue pressure on your neck and shoulders. Over time, it can leave you with a real pain in the neck! If you sleep in an awkward position with your head and shoulders propped up with lots of pillows, you are also at risk of hurting your neck. There is a simple solution: Reprogram your body so that good posture becomes second nature.

When you have achieved good posture, your body is in neutral alignment. Good posture is when all the components of your body are properly aligned from your eyes to your shoulders to your hips to your toes. Your head is held straight, not turned or tilted to one side. From the front, your shoulders, hips, and knees are of equal height. Your shoulder should be aligned with your hip, your knee aligned with your ankle. From the side, you should see the three natural curves of your back, in the neck, upper back, and lower back. From the back view, the little bumps in your spine should fall in a straight line down the center of your back. This posture stance is called neutral alignment. You will notice that when I describe an exercise that is performed in an upright position, I will often remind you to keep your body in neutral alignment.

Good posture is not stiff or uncomfortable, it is relaxed and natural. It actually feels a lot better than poor posture.

Poor posture exacts a steep toll on your body. When you have poor posture, the body's proper vertical position is out of alignment and the back's natural curves become distorted. There are two typical poor standing postures. The first is what I call the Slump; I call the second the Soldier. They're both bad but in different ways. The Slump is the more common of the two poor postures; in it, the head is placed in a forward position. The shoulders and the upper back are rounded, but the lower back is arched with the buttocks protruding. The chest is sunk in and flattened, and the tummy is sagging. Not only is the Slump as bad for your muscles as it is unattractive, but it can have a lasting negative impact on your health. The caved-in upper-body position can crowd your internal organs, making it harder for your heart and lungs to do their jobs.

People who slump when they are standing typically slump when they are sitting at their desk or in their car, which means that they spend most of their waking hours in this poor position.

Lean machine alert: Lean machines are especially prone to the Slump and have to be extra-careful about maintaining good posture.

The Soldier is a basic military pose in which the head and shoulder blades are tightly pulled back, the lower back is arched, and the knees are locked or straight. This rigid position minimizes your spinal cord's ability to be a shock absorber for the body, so every time you take a step, you put a great deal of stress on your knee joints.

Anyone can have good posture if they work at it. The first and most important step is to find your ideal posture and to try to maintain it throughout the day. In addition to doing a posture check before you do your workout, I recommend that you take a minute or two throughout the day to periodically recheck your posture to make sure that you are in correct alignment.

posture check

The Wall Check

This simple test helps you align your body in its natural, neutral alignment with the S curve.

1. Stand with the back of your head and your buttocks touching the wall, and your heels about six inches away from the baseboard.

2. With your hand, check the distance between your lower back and the wall and your neck and the wall. If you can get within an inch or two at the lower back and two inches at the neck, you are close to having excellent posture.

3. Walk away from the wall, close your eyes, and *feel* how good it is to have good posture. *Visualize* what good posture looks like. This will teach your body how to achieve good posture all the time.

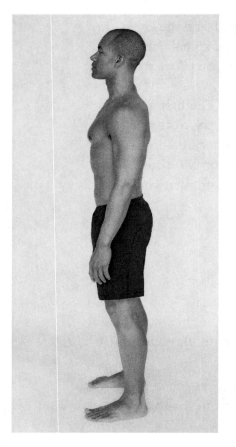

The Mirror Check

Stand forward facing a full-length mirror with your arms by your side. Check for the following:

1. Are your shoulders level? Make sure that one shoulder is not higher or lower than the other.

2. Is your head straight and not tilted to one side?

3. Are the spaces between your arms and your sides equal on both sides?

4. Are your hips level and your kneecaps facing straight ahead? Your knees should not be turned out to the side.

5. Are your ankles straight and not turned out to the side?

Turn to your right side, and check for the following. (If it is difficult for you to do a side-view check, I recommend that you get someone to take a photograph of you from the side and you can do your side-view check from this photo.)

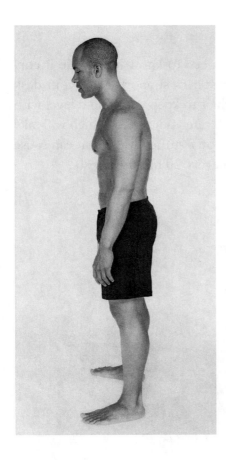

1. Is your head erect, not slumping forward or backwards?

2. Is your chin parallel to the floor, not tilting up or down?

3. Are your shoulders in line with your ears, not drooping forward or pulled back?

4. Is your stomach flat and not sagging?

5. Are both knees straight and not turned out to the side?

6. Does your lower back have a slightly forward curve—but not too flat or curved too forward, hollowing out your back in an unnatural way?

Turn to your left side, and repeat the test.

noble ways to improve your posture

standing

Check your posture throughout the day. When you are standing, be sure to hold your head high with your chin slightly tucked in, your shoulders gently back, your chest out (but not jutting out), and your stomach tucked in to improve your balance. If your job requires you to be on your feet all day, fatigue can often result in poor posture. You can take some pressure off your lower back by resting one foot on a footstool whenever you can. Take periodic breaks to sit down and try to keep this neutral alignment when you sit.

sitting

So much of our time is spent sitting, we need to know how to do it correctly. At work, use a chair with firm lower-back support. Keep your desk or table top elbow high, and adjust the chair to keep your knees level with your hips. You can also use a footrest to elevate your knees, which will take pressure off the back of the legs. Don't sit on a stuffed wallet—it can cause hip imbalances. Get up and walk around every 20 minutes or so.

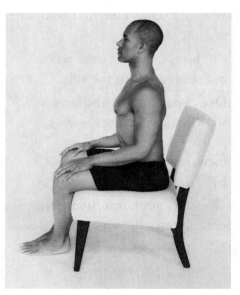 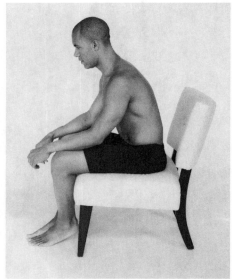

working in front of a computer screen

A poorly designed workplace is a recipe for neck strain, upper-back pain, eyestrain, arm and wrist problems, and even headaches. Keep your computer screen slightly below eye level (around 15 degrees). Place reference materials on a copy stand even with and close to the computer terminal. Never set the monitor off to one side so that you have to twist your neck in an unnatural and uncomfortable position. Every 20 minutes or so, get up from your desk and stretch your muscles. Invest in an ergonomic work chair designed to prevent injury. There are numerous ergonomic office chairs on the market; try out a few chairs before you invest in one. Comfort is very subjective, and what works for one person may not work for another.

sitting in your car

North Americans spend more time than ever before in their cars—on average, every North American drives around 14,000 miles a year, often in stifling traffic. Spending hours a day in a cramped, awkward position is bound to take its toll on your body. Be sure your car ride is as comfortable as possible. Adjust the seat forward so that your knees are level with your hips. Place a small pillow or cushion in the small of your back to prevent back strain.

sleeping

We spend around one-third of our lives in bed. The position you sleep in can have a tremendous impact on how you feel when you are awake. Even when you are lying down, maintain proper alignment. Buy high-quality bedding. A firm mattress will support the spine and help maintain good posture while you sleep. If you like to sleep on your side, lie with your knees bent and your head supported by a pillow. Be sure that your head is level with your spine, not propped way up out of alignment. If you prefer to sleep on your back, avoid using thick pillows under your head. Instead, use a small pillow under your neck. Don't sleep on your stomach, because it puts too much stress on your back muscles.

lifting

Lifting the wrong way can cause a real backache. Let your legs do the work to prevent injury to your lower back. Stand close to the object, then squat down and straddle it. Grasp the object and slowly lift the load by straightening your legs as you stand up. Don't twist from the waist. Rotating your spine while putting pressure on it can lead to muscle or ligament strain or even a herniated disk. Always point your toes in the direction your hands are moving. Carry the object close to your body so that you engage all of your muscles and avoid putting undue stress on any one muscle group such as your lower back.

bending

If you don't bend the right way, you can throw your back out. Never twist from the waist and bend over at the same time. It puts too much pressure on your spine. To lift or reach for something on the floor, bend your knees while keeping your back straight.

Tips for Lifelong Good Posture

- Excess weight, especially around the middle, pulls on the back, weakening your stomach muscles. Weak stomach muscles cannot provide enough support for the lower back, which is a major cause of back problems.
- Regular exercise keeps you flexible and helps strengthen your muscles so that they can support proper posture.
- Last but not least, be aware of your posture when you are standing, sitting, or lying down. Make posture checks a regular part of your day.

---

part two

the
body noble
workout

how to work out

your body noble home gym

With the Body Noble Workout, you don't need to invest a lot of money in fancy equipment that takes up space in your home and often ends up collecting dust. You can do my entire workout with just three basic pieces of equipment: an exercise ball (also called a Swiss ball, a core ball, a stability ball, or a balance ball), a set of exercise cables (also called resistance tubes), and an exercise mat or a thick towel. That's it. You can purchase the equipment at most discount stores (such as Wal-Mart, Kmart, Costco, or Sam's Club), at sporting goods stores, or even on the Internet. Your entire investment should be around $50. With these pieces of equipment, combined with a knowledge of how to properly engage and work your muscle groups, you can get an even better workout than you would at a gym filled with high-tech, expensive exercise machines.

Exercise Ball   An exercise ball is one of the most versatile pieces of exercise equipment ever invented. You can do virtually any kind of exercise on a ball, from sit-ups to pull-ups to push-ups. Working with an exercise ball adds an additional dimension to an exercise, forcing you to utilize muscles that build strength and promote balance. You

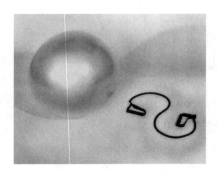

use more muscle groups when you work out with an exercise ball than you do using machines at the gym that typically isolate only one muscle group at a time! Even the simple act of just sitting on an exercise ball forces you to engage your core muscles to maintain your balance. Inflatable exercise balls are often sold deflated to save space in the store, or shipping costs. You should purchase an inflation pump with the ball so that you can blow the ball up easily (in many cases, it will come with a pump). Exercise balls deflate over time, so be sure to periodically pump in air to maintain the right degree of firmness. Exercise balls typically come in four sizes: 45 cm, or 18 inches, high; 55 cm, or 22 inches, high; 65 cm, or 26 inches, high; and 75 cm, or 30 inches, high. Pick the right size for you depending on your height. As a general rule, if you are under 5', you should use the 45 cm ball; if you are 5' to 5'6", you should use a 55 cm ball; if you are 5'7" to 6'0", you should use a 65 cm ball; and if you are 6'1" or taller, you should use a 75 cm ball.

Exercise Cable   An exercise cable is a long rubber tube with a handle on each end. Most of the exercises recommended in this book require a 4-foot-long cable. Exercise cables help build muscle by providing resistance, taking the place of weights and exercise machines. Exercise cables come in different strengths. Pick the right resistance level for you. There is no uniform method of measuring resistance; each brand has its own method. I generally advise moderately fit beginners to start with a cable that has moderate or medium resistance, and for more fit people to use a brand that has heavy resistance. Some brands offer extra-duty exercise cables for body builders and elite athletes, but unless you are very strong, I don't advise using them. Exercise cables are easy to use, but remember that they are like giant rubber bands. Be sure that they are securely attached to the body part you are working, so that when you stretch them, they don't snap off and hit you in the face.

You can buy exercise cables just about everywhere these days. Buy two sets of cables and keep one at the office so you can always do a quick workout.

Exercise Mat   You can lie on a towel if you like, but for a small investment, you can have a truly comfortable workout with an exercise or yoga mat. You can purchase a good mat for $30 or less. Be sure to get a mat that is thick enough to be comfortable but can be rolled up and stuck in a closet or under your bed.

Got your ball, your cables, and your mat? Now you're ready for your workout.

the body noble technique

Before you begin the Body Noble Workout, take two minutes to review the Noble Technique to prepare your body and mind for a terrific workout.

When I train people, I change the routine periodically to keep it fresh. That's why I sometimes offer two different exercise options for the same muscle group. I recommend that you alternate between these exercises every time you work out. In some cases, I offer a more advanced version of an exercise for those who may need a bit more of a challenge. After you exercise each muscle group, please stretch out your working muscles. This helps maintain flexibility, prevents injury, and improves the results of your workout.

When you first begin the program, it may take you slightly longer than 20 minutes, but once you become familiar with the exercises, you will move through the program quickly.

take a noble breath

Sit up tall on a chair or your exercise ball. Make sure that your back is straight and your shoulders are upright (not hunched forward). Put your hands on your stomach. Take a deep breath in through your nose and allow your stomach to expand as you breathe in. Count 1, 2, 3, 4 as you fill your stomach with air. Squeeze in your diaphragm muscles as you push the air out up toward your chest and out through your nose. Count 1, 2, 3, 4 as you exhale. Repeat 5 times. (This should take around 30 seconds.)

visualization

Continue to sit up tall and close your eyes. Visualize your body as you experience your favorite vacation. Continue your deep breathing. Feel your lower body fill up with air. Feel your breath travel from your abdomen to your legs to your toes. Feel your breath in your feet move up toward your ankles and your knees and into your lower back. Push your stomach up through your chest and out through your head. Feel a white light surrounding your healthy, beautiful body. Think to yourself, *I love my healthy beautiful body. I am strong and sexy. I am healthy. I love myself. I take good care of myself.* Now give yourself a hug. (This should take around 30 seconds.)

touch training

Do a quick review of the different muscle groups you will be working. Visualize each muscle group as you lightly touch it with your hands. Start with your abs. Move on to your chest . . . your biceps . . . your triceps . . . your shoulders . . . your back . . . your legs . . . your hamstrings . . . your butt . . . your calves. Squeeze each muscle and feel it contract. Go deep within yourself and feel the muscles that are at the core of your foundation. (This should take around 30 seconds.)

posture check

Stand up tall with your back against a flat wall. Position your feet shoulder width apart with your knees slightly bent and your abs slightly contracted. Your shoulders and back should be upright, your chin slightly tucked in, and your head facing forward.

Visualize a thin string being drawn down through your head, through the center of your body to the ground.

Step away from the wall and walk across the room. Let this neutral position permeate your body. Keep this perfect posture while you do your exercise routine and in your daily life. (This should take around 30 seconds.)

the body noble workout

Standard Abdominal Crunch

Advanced Abdominal Crunch

Oblique Crunch

Reverse Crunch

Advanced Reverse Crunch

Pelvic Tilt

Push-Up *or* Exercise Cable
  Chest Fly

Doorway Stretch

Exercise Cable Lat Pull-Down
  or Exercise Cable Mid-
  Back One-Arm Row

Mid-Back Stretch

Exercise Cable Shoulder Press
  or Exercise Cable Lat
  Raise

Shoulder Stretch

Exercise Cable Bicep Curl

Bicep Stretch

Exercise Cable Tricep
  Kickback

Tricep Stretch

Exercise Ball Leg Extension

Exercise Ball Hamstring Curl

Exercise Ball Leg Squat
  or Exercise Ball Wall Squat
  or Partner Ball Squat
  or Exercise Cable Squat

Quad Stretch

Exercise Ball Butt Stretch

Exercise Cable Side Leg Raise
  or Exercise Ball Inner-
  Thigh Squeeze

Exercise Cable Calf Raise

Hamstring Stretch

Back Extension

Lower-Back Butt Stretch

Lower-Back Stretch

Standard Abdominal Crunch

I begin the Body Noble Workout with a series of abdominal strengthening exercises. I consider abs to be so important, I put them first. If you don't have time to do anything else, be sure to do your abs! Strong abs provide the foundation for a stable, fit body. When your abs are weak, you are prone to poor posture and joint problems, especially hip and back problems. You are also more likely to have poor balance later in life. All competitive sports, from tennis to golf to race car driving, rely on a strong midsection to hold the body securely in place. All of life's activities, from walking to running to bending down and picking up a child, depend on a stable midsection. Keep those abs strong. For the abdominal exercises, everyone should work up to 15 to 20 repetitions of your body type.

Equipment needed: Towel or mat

Working muscles: Abdominals

1. Lie flat on your back on a mat or towel with your knees bent. Place your hands under your head with your fingertips lightly touching each other. Visualize that you have a tennis ball tucked under your chin. This prevents you from letting your chin drop down to your chest, which puts a strain on your upper back and neck.

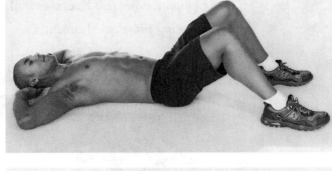

2. Crunch upward as you shorten the space between your chest and pelvis. Move up on a count of 1, 2. Hold the contraction and feel your ab muscles as you squeeze at the end range.

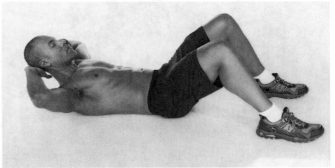

3. Move down on a count of 1, 2, 3, 4. Visualize a water balloon in your abdominal area. As you do the exercise, squeeze your ab muscles as if you were trying to compress the balloon and wring out all the water. You are using your own body weight to create resistance. Don't let gravity take over—keep working those ab muscles.

Lean Machine   Do two sets, 15 to 20 repetitions per set.

Muscle Maker   Do two sets, 15 to 20 repetitions per set.

Fat Fighter   Do two sets, 15 to 20 repetitions per set.

Advanced Abdominal Crunch

When the Standard Crunch becomes too easy, try this exercise. The addition of the exercise ball makes the standard ab crunch harder by creating additional stress on your midsection core muscles.

Equipment needed: Exercise ball

Working muscles: Abdominals

1. Lie flat on the exercise ball with your feet shoulder width apart and your head supported by your hands. Keep your chin up.

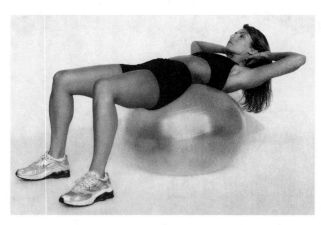

2. Crunch upward as you shorten the space between your chest and pelvis. Move up on a count of 1, 2. Hold the contraction and feel your ab muscles as you squeeze at the end range.

3. Move down on a count of 1, 2, 3, 4. Visualize a water balloon in your abdominal area. As you do the exercise, squeeze your ab muscles as if you were trying to compress the balloon and squeeze out all the water. You are using your own body weight to create resistance. Don't let gravity take over—keep working those ab muscles.

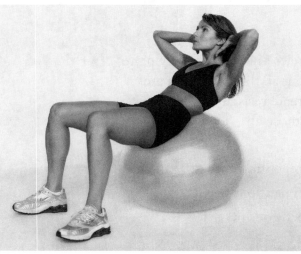

Lean Machine   Do two sets, 15 to 20 repetitions per set.

Muscle Maker   Do two sets, 15 to 20 repetitions per set.

Fat Fighter   Do two sets, 15 to 20 repetitions per set.

Oblique Crunch *(Left Side-Right Side)*

If you are pressed for time, you can do the Oblique Crunch one day and the Reverse Crunch the next time you work out.

Equipment needed: Towel or mat

Working muscles: Obliques

1. Lie flat on your back on a mat or towel with your legs rotated to your right side. Place your hands under your head. Keep your chin up.

2. Crunch upward but slightly turn toward your right knee as you come up.

3. Move up and to the side for a count of 1, 2 and down to starting position to a count of 1, 2, 3, 4.

4. Do 1 full set on your right side. Switch to your left side. Repeat.

Lean Machine   Do two sets, 15 to 20 repetitions per set.

Muscle Maker   Do two sets, 15 to 20 repetitions per set.

Fat Fighter   Do two sets, 15 to 20 repetitions per set.

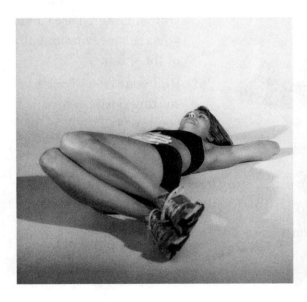 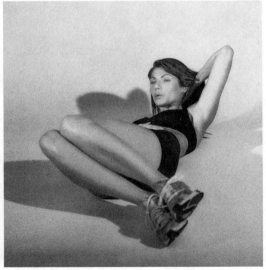

Reverse Crunch

If you are pressed for time, you can do the Reverse Crunch one day and the Oblique Crunch the next time you work out.

Equipment needed: Towel or mat

Working muscles: Lower abdominal area

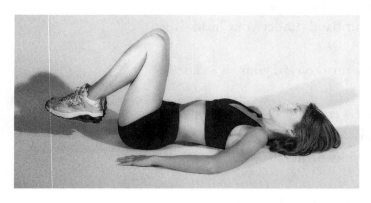

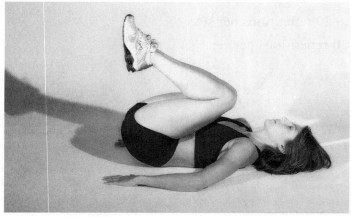

1. Lie flat on the floor on a mat or towel with your knees bent. Place your hands flat on the floor and at the side of your hips.

2. Roll your knees in toward your chest for a count of 1, 2. Place one hand on your lower abs. Feel the contraction in your lower abs. Visualize that you have an imaginary water balloon in your abdominal area and you are squeezing out all of the water.

3. Roll your knees back to starting position for a count of 1, 2, 3, 4.

Lean Machine Do two sets, 15 to 20 repetitions per set.

Muscle Maker Do two sets, 15 to 20 repetitions per set.

Fat Fighter Do two sets, 15 to 20 repetitions per set.

Advanced Reverse Crunch

With the addition of the ball, you need to use a lot more of your stabilizing muscles to bring the ball into your chest.

Equipment needed: Exercise ball

Working muscles: Lower abdominals

1. Lie flat on the floor with your knees bent 90 degrees resting on the ball. Stabilize the ball with the back of your legs.

2. Contract your heels into the ball and squeeze the ball with the back of your legs as you roll the ball in toward your chest. Remember to exhale on exertion and inhale at rest.

3. Bring the ball back to the starting position.

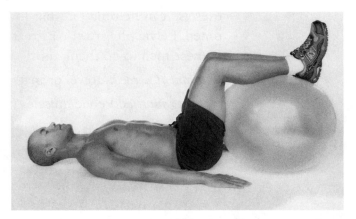

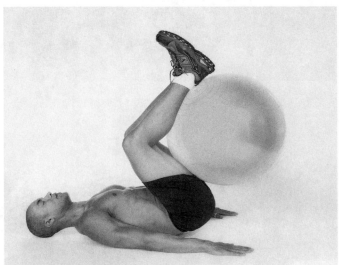

Lean Machine   Do two sets, 15 to 20 repetitions per set.

Muscle Maker   Do two sets, 15 to 20 repetitions per set.

Fat Fighter   Do two sets, 15 to 20 repetitions per set.

Pelvic Tilt

Your pelvic muscles are deep within your body—you can't really see them, but you can certainly feel them. A common complaint among my women clients is that they think they're bloated, or retaining fluid. The truth is, many women do not have well-toned pelvic muscles, which creates a slight bulge below their abs. This pelvic tilt exercise can help flatten that lower ab area and make it feel more toned. Pelvic tilts are also a great exercise for the entire midriff, and I advise men to do them, too.

Equipment needed: Towel or mat

Working muscles: Pelvic muscles (right below your belly button)

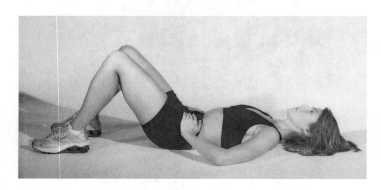

1. Lie flat on the floor with your feet shoulder width apart and your hands placed below your belly button.

2. Flex your pelvis upward as you squeeze your muscles in your lower pelvic area. Hold the squeeze and exhale on the contraction. This is a subtle movement involving your pelvic muscles. It's easy to let your glutes do the work, but don't.

Lean Machine   Do two sets, 15 to 20 repetitions per set.

Muscle Maker   Do two sets, 15 to 20 repetitions per set.

Fat Fighter   Do two sets, 15 to 20 repetitions per set.

Push-Up

You can alternate between the Push-Up and the Exercise Cable Chest Fly. You can do push-ups on the floor, on a couch, or on a bed as long as the mattress is firm.

Equipment needed: Towel or mat

Working muscles: Chest, arms, and shoulders

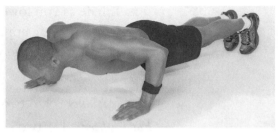

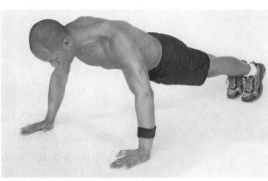

1. Lie flat, face down on a mat or towel on the floor with your hands shoulder width apart and your elbows bent 90 degrees. If you are a beginner, modify the push-up by keeping your knees slightly bent. If you are more advanced, keep your feet straight and try to keep your knees straight, but don't lock the knee joints. Make sure that your abs are contracted and your spine is in a neutral position.

2. Exhale as you push your body up. Keep the tension on your chest, upper-arm, and shoulder muscles. Use your body weight to create the resistance to tone your upper-body muscles. Count 1, 2 up.

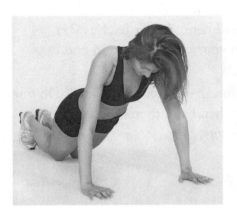

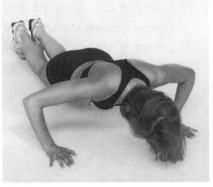

3. Inhale as you lower your body to a count of 1, 2, 3, 4, still working your upper body. Don't allow momentum to bring you down, do the work!

Lean Machine   Do two sets, 8 to 10 repetitions per set.

Muscle Maker   Do two sets, 10 to 15 repetitions per set.

Fat Fighter   Do two sets, 15 to 20 repetitions per set.

Exercise Cable Chest Fly

This exercise gives your chest more definition. Well-formed inner-chest muscles can create the illusion of cleavage in a natural, healthy way. You can alternate between the Exercise Cable Chest Fly and the Push-Up.

Equipment needed: Exercise cable

Working muscles: Chest, inner chest, and shoulders

1. Stand up tall in your neutral alignment. Stand on one end of the exercise cable with both feet and let the cable handle stay on the floor. Hold the other cable handle in your right hand, and start with both arms at your side.

2. Without bending your arm, use your right hand to pull the handle up to the height of the midsection of your chest to a count of 1, 2. Imagine a board behind your back as you squeeze down the middle of your chest. Maintain good posture!

3. Return to the starting position to a count of 1, 2, 3, 4. Do one complete set with your right hand and then one complete set with your left hand. Do two sets.

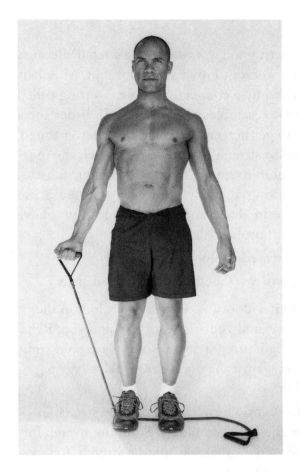

Lean Machine   Do two sets, 8 to 10 repetitions per set.

Muscle Maker   Do two sets, 10 to 15 repetitions per set.

Fat Fighter   Do two sets, 15 to 20 repetitions per set.

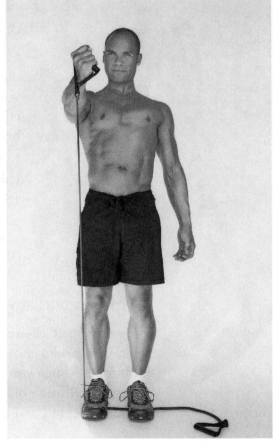

Doorway Stretch

Why do I interrupt a perfectly good workout with a stretch? Because stretching can turn a good workout into a great workout. Muscle is

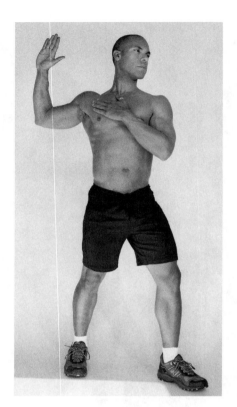

surrounded by a connective tissue covering called fascia that resembles plastic wrap. In order for a muscle to get bigger and, ultimately, better toned, you have to stretch out the fascia so that the muscle has room to grow. If you stretch your muscles after working them, you're going to see a big difference in shape and tone. (Avoid if you have rotator cuff problems.)

Equipment needed: Doorway

Working muscles: Chest, shoulders, and arms

1. Stand in a doorway. Put your left foot in the doorway and your right foot behind you. Bend your right arm 90 degrees and place your right elbow against the door frame. Take a deep breath.

2. Lean slightly forward and feel the stretch in your chest and shoulders. Hold the stretch for 15 seconds. Exhale during the stretch. Repeat on the other side.

Exercise Cable Lat Pull-Down

When my male clients tell me they want that cut, inverted-triangle look, with broad shoulders and a slim waist, I recommend the lat pull-down. When you increase the size and tone of your lat muscles, it gives the illusion of a smaller waist. You can alternate between the Exercise Cable Lat Pull-Down and the Exercise Cable Mid-Back Row.

Equipment needed: Exercise cable

Working muscles: Lats and biceps

1. Stand in neutral alignment with your feet about shoulder width apart and your knees slightly bent. Hold the exercise cable in both of your hands and place it above your head.

2. Pull the cable with both hands as you bend one arm and bring the band down and in toward your side to a count of 1, 2. Continue to pull the band apart as you bring it down. This will isolate your back muscles.

3. Bring the cable back over your head to the starting position to a count of 1, 2, 3, 4.

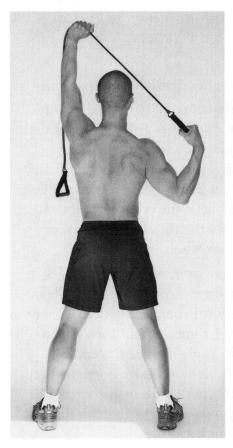 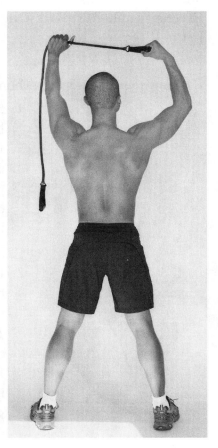

4. Repeat the exercise with your alternate hand and arm to the other side.

Lean Machine   Do two sets, 8 to 10 repetitions per set.

Muscle Maker   Do two sets, 10 to 15 repetitions per set.

Fat Fighter   Do two sets, 15 to 20 repetitions per set.

Exercise Cable Mid-Back One-Arm Row

This exercise does so much in so little time! Strengthening the mid-back is a great way to prevent shoulder and neck problems. It also promotes good posture and balance. You can alternate between the Exercise Cable Mid-Back One-Arm Row and the Exercise Cable Lat Pull-Down.

Equipment needed: Exercise cable

Working muscles: Mid-back rhomboids, deltoids, and trapezius

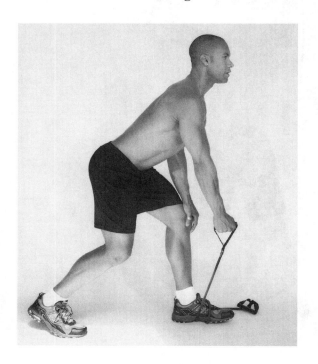

1. Stand up tall in neutral alignment but lean forward from the waist. Imagine that you are skiing on air. Keep your back straight and your chest up. Wrap the exercise cable around your left foot and hold the right handle in your right hand.

2. Lean over, but keep your back neutral. Row the right handle in toward your mid-back to a count of 1, 2. Squeeze your back as you roll the cable in toward your back. Hold the squeeze. Focus on keeping your elbow in at your side as you contract the muscles through your back.

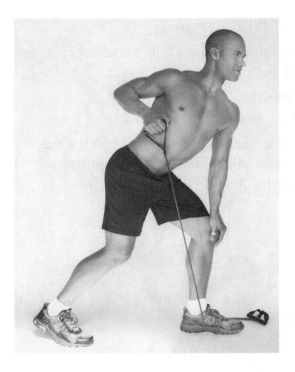

3. Return to the starting position to a count of 1, 2, 3, 4. Repeat on your left side.

Lean Machine   Do two sets, 8 to 10 repetitions per set.

Muscle Maker   Do two sets, 10 to 15 repetitions per set.

Fat Fighter   Do two sets, 15 to 20 repetitions per set.

Mid-Back Stretch

We need to stretch out our muscles more often. Do this stretch several times a day. It's like giving your body a reward for all its hard work.

Equipment needed: None

Working muscles: Mid-back, neck, and arms

1. Stand up tall in neutral alignment with your feet shoulder width apart. Fully extend your arms in front of you. Place your right hand over your left hand.

2. Inhale as you contract your abs inward. Exhale as you stretch through your mid-back. Feel the stretch in your upper back and neck muscles. Hold the stretch for 15 seconds.

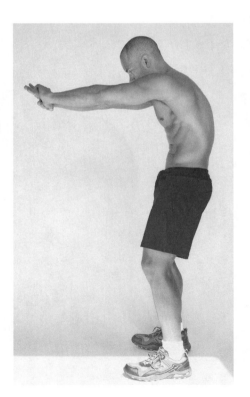

Exercise Cable Shoulder Press

You can alternate between the Exercise Cable Shoulder Press and the Exercise Cable Lat Raise

Equipment needed: Exercise cable

Working muscles: Shoulders, deltoids, and triceps

1. Place your feet shoulder width apart and stand on the exercise cable holding the handles in both hands. Your hands should be at shoulder height.

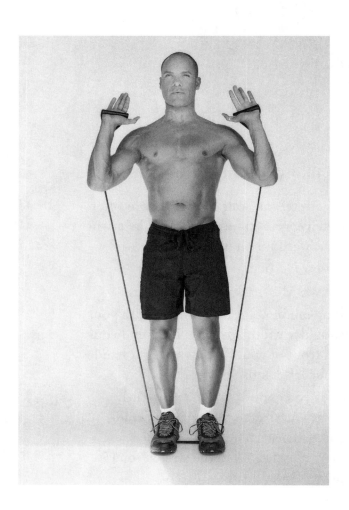

2. With both hands, pull the handles over your head to a count of 1, 2. Do not lock your elbows. Feel the squeeze in your shoulder muscles.

3. Lower the handles to starting position to a count of 1, 2, 3, 4.

Lean Machine   Do two sets, 8 to 10 repetitions per set.

Muscle Maker   Do two sets, 10 to 15 repetitions per set.

Fat Fighter   Do two sets, 15 to 20 repetitions per set.

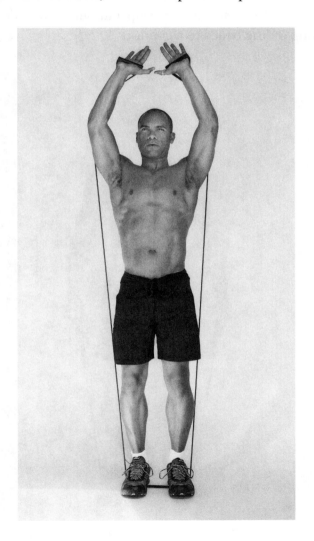

Exercise Cable Lat Raise

You can alternate between the Exercise Cable Lat Raise and the Exercise Cable Shoulder Press.

Equipment needed: Exercise cable

Working muscles: Deltoids

1. Stand on the exercise cable and hold one handle in each hand, with your arms at your sides.

2. Standing tall, raise your arms up and out to the side while pulling on the bands to a count of 1, 2. Stop before you get as

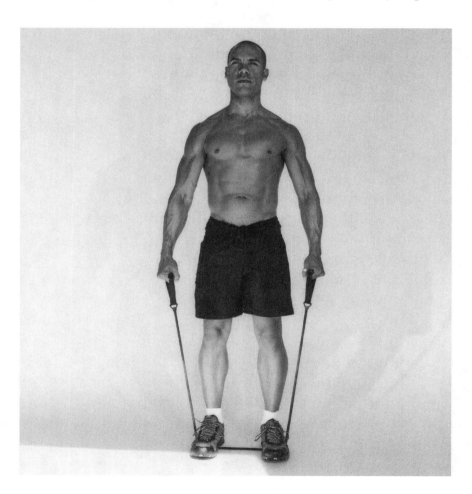

high as your ears or you will place too much stress on your shoulder joint.

3. Return to the starting position while maintaining your resistance, to a count of 1, 2, 3, 4. (Use one cable at a time if you are a beginner.)

Lean Machine   Do two sets, 8 to 10 repetitions per set.

Muscle Maker   Do two sets, 10 to 15 repetitions per set.

Fat Fighter   Do two sets, 15 to 20 repetitions per set.

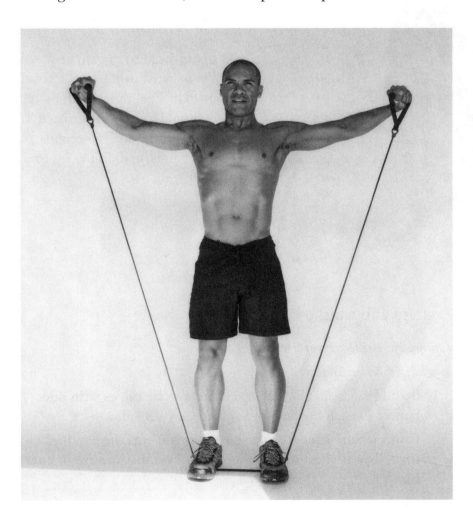

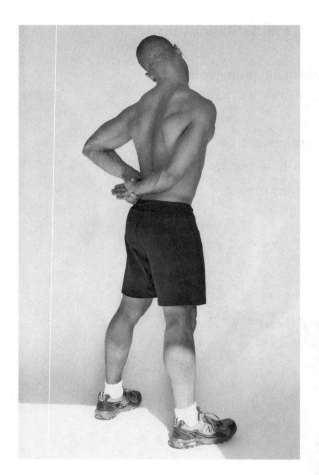

Shoulder Stretch

Tired of sitting at your desk? This is a great exercise for the office. Do it a few times a day.

Equipment needed: None

Working muscles: Deltoids

1. Stand up tall with your hands at your side. Take your left hand and grab your right wrist behind your back.

2. Tilt your head to the left as you pull your wrist to the left, across your body. Feel the stretch in your shoulders and upper back and neck. Hold for 15 seconds. Switch hands, and do the other side.

Exercise Cable Bicep Curl

Equipment needed: Exercise cable

Working muscles: Biceps

1. Stand in neutral alignment on the exercise cables with one handle in each hand and your arms at your sides.

2. Contract and squeeze your biceps as you curl the handles toward your chest to a count of 1, 2. Feel the squeeze in your biceps.

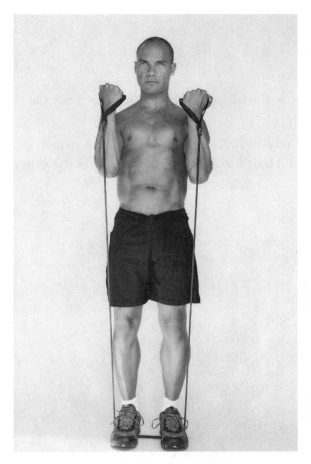

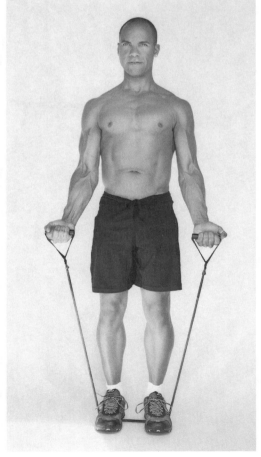

3. Return to your starting position while maintaining your resistance to a count of 1, 2, 3, 4.

Lean Machine Do two sets, 8 to 10 repetitions per set.

Muscle Maker Do two sets, 10 to 15 repetitions per set.

Fat Fighter Do two sets, 15 to 20 repetitions per set.

Bicep Stretch

Equipment needed: Wall

Working muscles: Biceps

1. Stand tall next to a wall with your arm and hand against the wall at chest height.

2. As you turn your body away from the wall, feel the stretch in your bicep muscles. Hold for 15 seconds. Repeat on the other side.

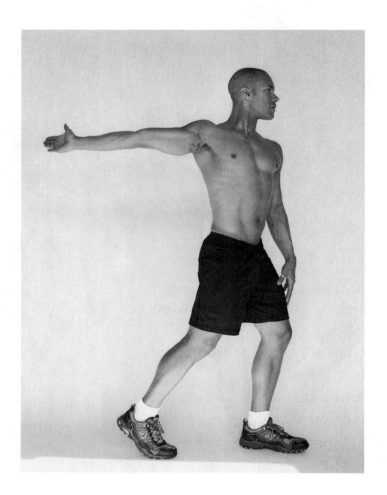

Exercise Cable Tricep Kickback

Equipment needed: Exercise cable

Working muscles: Triceps

1. Stand tall with your left foot on the exercise cable, holding a handle in your right hand.

2. Lean over at your waist while extending your elbow backward but keeping your arm close to your body to a count of 1, 2. Feel the contraction in the back of your arm.

3. Return to starting position to a count of 1, 2, 3, 4. Repeat on the other side.

Lean Machine   Do two sets, 8 to 10 repetitions per set.

Muscle Maker   Do two sets, 10 to 15 repetitions per set.

Fat Fighter   Do two sets, 15 to 20 repetitions per set.

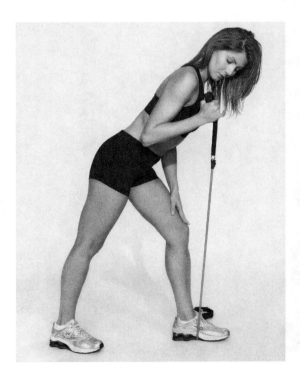
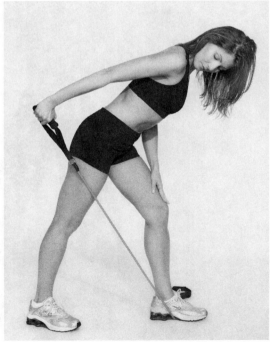

Tricep Stretch

Equipment needed: None

Working muscles: Triceps

1. Stand in neutral alignment with your feet shoulder width apart.

2. Place your right arm at the side of your head and grab your right elbow with your left hand, and pull toward the top of your head.

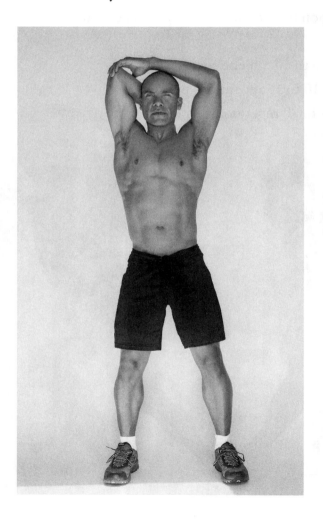

3. Feel the stretch in your right tricep. Hold the stretch for 15 seconds.

4. Switch arms and repeat the stretch.

Exercise Ball Leg Extension
(Left Leg, Right Leg)

This is a great exercise for balance.

Equipment needed: Exercise ball

Working muscles: Quads

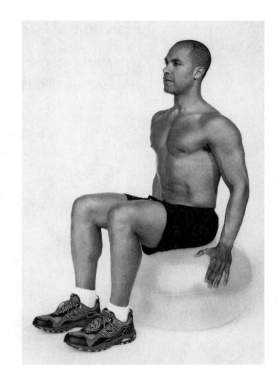

1. Sit up tall on the exercise ball with both feet in front of you. Place your hands on the ball if you need help staying balanced. (As you become more advanced, you should be able to do this exercise without the assistance of your arms.)

2. Extend your left leg to a count of 1, 2. Focus on isolating your left front thigh quadriceps muscle. Imagine that you are moving your leg through quicksand. You have to work hard against resistance. Feel the squeeze.

3. Continue to squeeze as you lower your left leg to the starting position to a count of 1, 2, 3, 4. Switch legs and repeat the exercise. Do one complete set on your left leg before switching to your right leg.

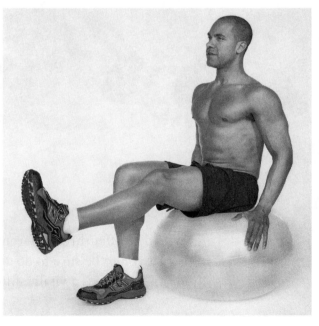

Lean Machine Do two sets, 8 to 10 repetitions per set.

Muscle Maker Do two sets, 10 to 15 repetitions per set.

Fat Fighter Do two sets, 15 to 20 repetitions per set.

Exercise Ball Hamstring Curl

Equipment needed: Exercise ball
Working muscles: Hamstrings and calves

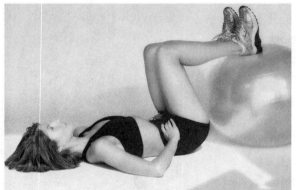

1. Lie flat on your back on the floor with the heels of both feet firmly planted on the ball.

2. Press your heels firmly down on the ball. Touch the back of your calves with the ball. Roll the ball in toward your glutes as you squeeze your leg muscles to a count of 1, 2. Return to starting position.

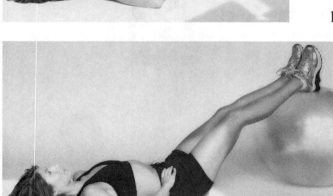

3. Roll the ball back out to a count of 1, 2, 3, 4.

Lean Machine   Do two sets, 8 to 10 repetitions per set.

Muscle Maker   Do two sets, 10 to 15 repetitions per set.

Fat Fighter   Do two sets, 15 to 20 repetitions per set.

Exercise Ball Leg Squat

Why do I offer three different exercises for the basic squat? Because I want you to be sure to do at least one of them each time you work out. Squatting is a vitally important movement for everyday activities. Every time you get up and down from a chair or go from a kneeling to a standing position, you are doing a squat. To maintain stability, you need strong leg muscles and glutes. If you are weak in your legs and glutes, you will be more prone to back, hip, and knee injuries. You can prevent a lot of problems down the road if you are vigilant about doing your squats. You can alternate between the Exercise Ball Leg Squat, the Exercise Ball Wall Squat, and the Exercise Cable Squat.

Equipment needed: Exercise ball

Working muscles: Glutes, quads, hamstrings, and adductors

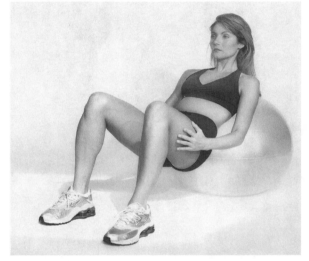

1. Sit on the exercise ball with both feet in front of you. Roll down and press against the ball with your lower back. Your feet should be in front of the ball shoulder width apart.

2. Squeeze the back of your legs and hamstring muscles as you roll up on the ball to a count of 1, 2. Focus on contracting your legs.

3. Roll back down to a count of 1, 2, 3, 4, still fully engaging your leg muscles.

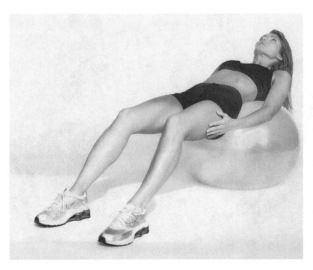

Lean Machine   Do two sets, 8 to 10 repetitions per set.

Muscle Maker   Do two sets, 10 to 15 repetitions per set.

Fat Fighter   Do two sets, 15 to 20 repetitions per set.

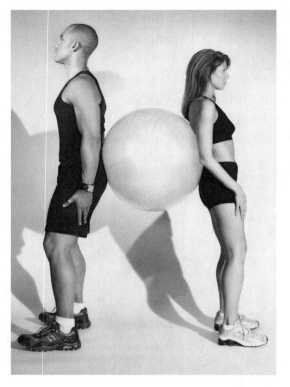

Exercise Ball Wall Squat or Partner Ball Squat

You can alternate between the Exercise Ball Leg Squat, the Exercise Cable Squat, and the Exercise Ball Wall Squat.

Equipment needed: Exercise ball and wall or partner

Working muscles: Quads, hamstrings, and glutes

1. Place an exercise ball against the wall and hold the ball in place by pressing against it with the lower part of your back, your lordotic curve. Your feet should be shoulder width apart. (Or you can do this exercise with a friend.)

2. Push your lower back into the ball. Roll down and bend your knees 90 degrees. Keep your feet pointing forward, pushing off from your heels. You will feel the work in your butt and thighs.

3. Roll your body back up to the starting position to a count of 1, 2, 3, 4.

Lean Machine   Do two sets, 8 to 10 repetitions per set.

Muscle Maker   Do two sets, 10 to 15 repetitions per set.

Fat Fighter   Do two sets, 15 to 20 repetitions per set.

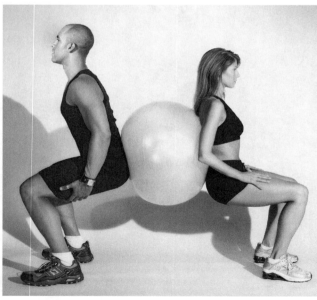

Exercise Cable Squat

You can alternate between the Exercise Ball Leg Squat, the Exercise Ball Wall Squat, and the Exercise Cable Squat.

Equipment needed: Exercise cable

Working muscles: Quads, glutes, and hamstrings

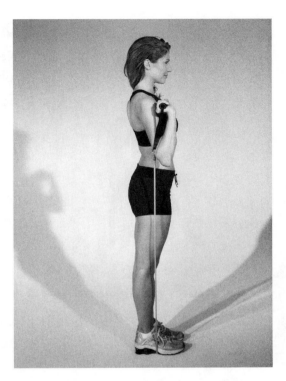

1. Stand with both feet on the cable, shoulder width apart. Hold one cable handle in each hand at shoulder height and keep your shoulders level and your elbows at your sides. Be sure to maintain good posture.

2. Bend your legs 90 degrees and sit back while squeezing your butt and lower leg muscles. Hold the cables firmly in your hands and be sure to keep them at shoulder height and your shoulders level. Your knees should not go past your toes. Keep your back straight and don't round your shoulders.

3. Return to the starting position.

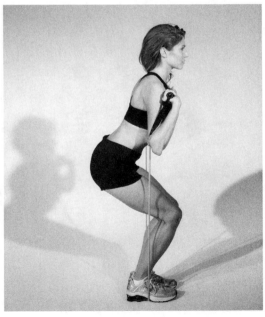

Lean Machine Do two sets, 8 to 10 repetitions per set.

Muscle Maker Do two sets, 10 to 15 repetitions per set.

Fat Fighter Do two sets, 15 to 20 repetitions per set.

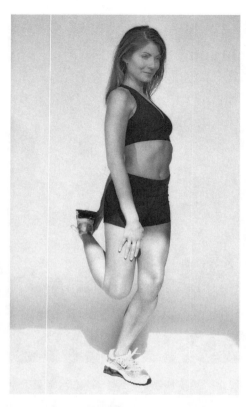

Quad Stretch

Keeping your quads strong and flexible goes a long way to preventing knee injuries.

Equipment needed: None

Working muscles: Quads

1. Stand in neutral position with your feet shoulder width apart.

2. Grab your right ankle with your left hand as you flex your knee back and stretch the front of your right thigh. Keep the knee aligned with the opposite leg. Hold the stretch for 15 seconds.

3. Return to the starting position and stretch your left thigh.

Exercise Ball Butt Stretch

This exercise is good for people who have sciatica, an irritation of the sciatic nerve that can result in lower-back pain radiating down from the buttocks. It helps prevent the glutes from getting tight, which can trigger even more pain in that area.

Equipment needed: Exercise ball

Working muscles: Glutes

1. Sit up tall on the exercise ball. Bend your right leg and place it over your left thigh.

2. Lean over and feel the stretch in your right glutes (butt). Hold the stretch for 15 seconds. Repeat on the other side.

Exercise Cable Side Leg Raise

This exercise is great for balance. You can alternate the Exercise Cable Side Leg Raise with the Exercise Ball Inner-Thigh Squeeze.

Equipment needed: Exercise cable

Working muscles: Sides, glutes, and hips

1. Stand on an exercise cable with your legs shoulder width apart with one handle in each hand.

2. Extend one leg out to the side to a count of 1, 2, allowing the band to create resistance against your foot. Feel the squeeze on your outer thigh muscles.

3. Return to the starting position to a count of 1, 2, 3, 4 while maintaining resistance.

Lean Machine   Do two sets, 8 to 10 repetitions per set.

Muscle Maker   Do two sets, 10 to 15 repetitions per set.

Fat Fighter   Do two sets, 15 to 20 repetitions per set.

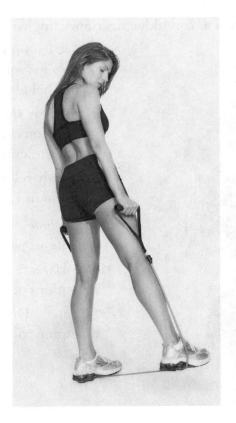 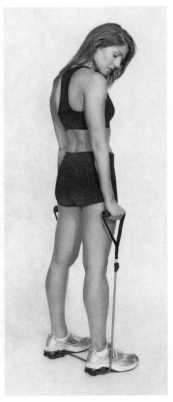

Exercise Ball Inner-Thigh Squeeze

Your inner and outer thigh muscles help stabilize your pelvis, which balances your entire lower body. Women often ask me if doing this and other thigh exercises can make their thighs thinner. The answer is no. You can exercise your thighs until you are blue in the face and it may help give them better tone, but it won't make them thinner. There's no such thing as spot reducing, whether it's your thighs, your abs, or your butt. If you need to lean down, you have to add some cardio to your workout routine (see chapter 8), as well as do resistance training, and eat a "clean" diet. If you do those three things, you will see good results. You can alternate between the Exercise Cable Side Leg Raise and the Exercise Ball Inner-Thigh Squeeze.

Equipment needed: Exercise ball

Working muscles: Adductors (inner thighs) and abs

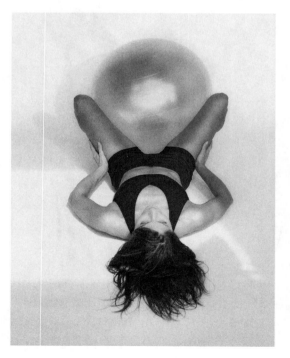

1. Lie flat on your back on the floor on a mat or towel with the exercise ball held between your legs.

2. Squeeze the ball with both legs and focus on contracting your abs during this exercise for a count of 1, 2.

3. Slowly release the squeeze to a count of 1, 2, 3, 4.

Lean Machine　Do two sets, 8 to 10 repetitions per set.

Muscle Maker　Do two sets, 10 to 15 repetitions per set.

Fat Fighter　Do two sets, 15 to 20 repetitions per set.

Exercise Cable Calf Raise

This exercise helps create more shapely calves, as well as strengthening the Achilles tendon, which helps stabilize your ankle area. If you have weak ankles, keep doing your calf raises.

Equipment needed: Exercise cable

Working muscles: Calves

1. Stand on the floor with your feet shoulder width apart, placing the cables under the soles of your feet and wrapping both handles around your hands.

2. Pull on the cables as you raise yourself up on the tips of your toes and contract your calf muscles to a count of 1, 2. Visualize that you are standing in quicksand and have to push your way out.

3. Hold the contraction at the top on your toes and slowly release to the starting position to a count of 1, 2, 3, 4.

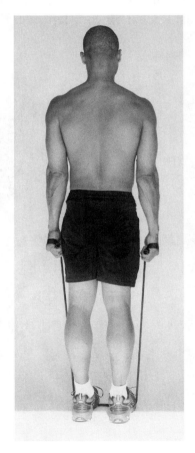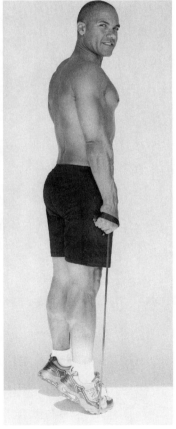

Lean Machine   Do two sets, 8 to 10 repetitions per set.

Muscle Maker   Do two sets, 10 to 15 repetitions per set.

Fat Fighter   Do two sets, 15 to 20 repetitions per set.

Hamstring Stretch

Tight hamstrings are a major cause of lower-back pain. Try to keep your hamstrings flexible, particularly as you get older.

Equipment needed: Exercise ball

Working muscles: Hamstrings and calves

1. Sit up tall on your exercise ball with the heel of your right foot on the ground about 1 foot in front of you and your left foot flat on the floor.

2. Lean forward from your waist and feel the stretch in the back of your right leg. Keep your back in a neutral alignment (don't hunch your shoulders). Hold the stretch for 15 seconds. Repeat on your left side. Exhale during the stretch.

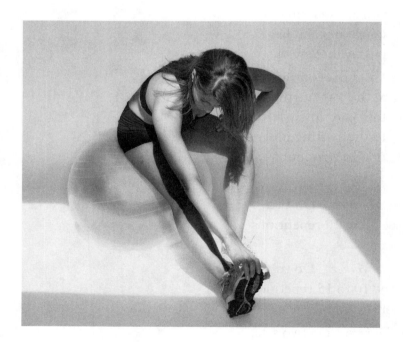

Back Extension

Equipment needed: Exercise ball

Muscles worked: Lower back and spinal muscles

1. Lie face down on your stomach on your exercise ball with your feet extended. Put both hands on the ball for balance.

2. Raise your head and chest, keeping your back in neutral alignment (don't arch your back) and hold for a count of 1, 2. Squeeze your back muscles as you extend your back. Working against resistance, return to your starting position. Hold for a count of 1, 2.

Lean Machine Do two sets, 8 to 10 repetitions per set.

Muscle Maker Do two sets, 10 to 15 repetitions per set.

Fat Fighter Do two sets, 15 to 20 repetitions per set.

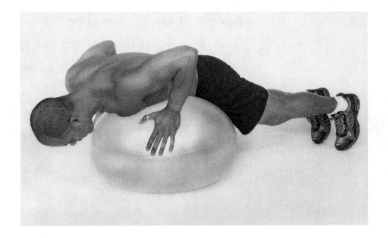

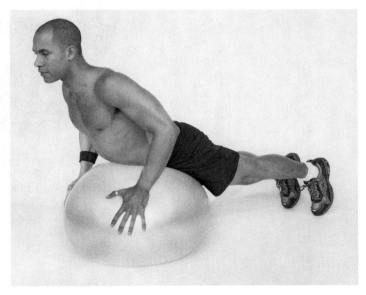

Lower-Back Butt Stretch

If you wake up with a stiff back, do this stretch before you even get out of bed in the morning. I do, and it helps to keep me flexible and pain free.

Equipment needed: Towel or mat

Working muscles: Lower back and glutes

1. Lie flat on your back on a mat, towel, or bed.

2. Bring both knees in toward your chest and place your arms around your knees. Feel the stretch in your back and glutes. Hold for 15 seconds. Exhale during the stretch.

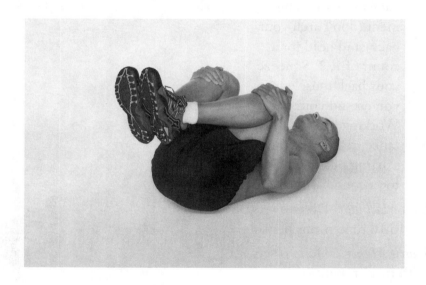

Lower-Back Stretch

Equipment needed: Towel or mat

Muscles worked: Lower back, glutes, and spinal muscles

1. Lie flat on the floor on your back on a mat or towel. Bring your left leg on top of your right thigh.

2. Roll your left knee down toward the floor with your right hand as you turn your head toward the left. Feel the stretch in your left lower back and glutes. Hold the stretch for 15 seconds. Exhale during the stretch.

3. Switch your legs and repeat the stretch.

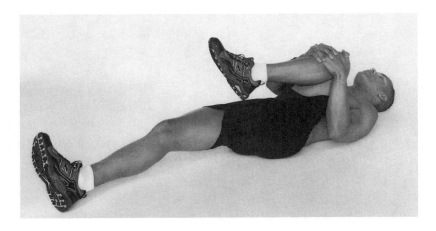

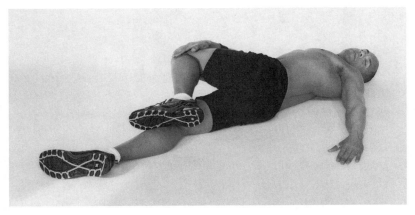

8

take a
cardio break

Whatever your body type, you need to do some kind of cardio-vascular exercise—cardio for short. Cardiovascular exercise (also called aerobics) describes any exercise that elevates your heart rate for a sustained period while utilizing oxygen. When done correctly, cardio trains your heart and lungs to pump blood more efficiently. Cardio is not just good for your body, it's also good for your spirit. It can be a lot of fun—for many people, their cardio breaks are the highlight of their days.

The heart is a muscle, and like any other muscle it needs to be exercised to stay fit. When you are sedentary, your heartbeat slows down. When you walk quickly, run, or ride a bicycle, your heartbeat increases. Your metabolism speeds up, and that promotes fat burning. Your heart and lungs must work harder to meet the increased demand for oxygen. The more you exercise, the more your heart and lungs become accustomed to the increased workload. Your heart will be able to do more work with less effort. You will develop more stamina, which means you will be able to walk or run for longer periods of time and not feel tired.

Why is this so important? If a well-conditioned heart is suddenly called upon to do extra work—let's say you have to run for a bus or walk up a few flights of steps—your heart should be able to meet the challenge. Your blood pressure will rise quickly as your heart pumps more blood, but it will return to normal as soon as you slow down. If your heart is not conditioned, however, your heart will not recover as quickly from the extra work. Your blood pressure will remain elevated, which will put added pressure on your heart. Over time, elevated blood pressure can cause damage to the arteries delivering blood to your heart, and this can result in heart attack and stroke. If you tire easily after exertion, you are less likely to exercise, and it becomes a vicious cycle. If you don't exercise your heart, when you do try to do some activity, you get so tired that you may stop. Over time, inactivity can destroy your heart and, in the long run, kill you. In the short run, you are going to miss out on a lot of good times because you're going to feel tired.

My point is, cardio is important. Make time for it. I have found that many people who follow resistance- or strength-training programs often skip cardio because they don't think they have the time to do both. Fortunately, it's much easier to fit cardio into your life than you may think. At one time, it was believed that you needed to do a full 30 minutes of cardio at one time to get any benefit. We now know that as long as you achieve 30 minutes of cardio daily, you can do it in intervals as short as 10 minutes at a time. I don't know anyone who can't find a spare 10 minutes two or three times a day.

For cardio to be effective, you must do it at the right level of intensity. It should be challenging enough to give your heart and lungs a good workout, but not so difficult that you are overtaxing your heart. That's why it's so important to work at your *target heart rate* or training level. Your target heart rate is the number of times your heart should beat per minute while you are working out. There's an easy formula that can help you find your target heart rate, which I share below.

1. Subtract your age from 220.

2. If you are beginning a fitness program, multiply that number by 60 percent. If you have been working out and are reasonably fit, multiply that number by 70 to 80 percent.

That's your target heart rate. The beginner will be working out at a slightly less intense level than the more experienced exerciser.

For example, if you are a forty-year-old who is just embarking on a cardio program, this is how you determine your target heart rate.

$$220 - 40 = 180$$
$$180 \times .60 = 128$$

Your target heart rate is 128.

How do you keep track of your target heart rate? You can measure it manually by taking your pulse for 10 seconds about 5 minutes into your cardio workout. By that time, you should be warmed up and your heart working at its training level. Multiply that number by 6 to find out how fast your heart is beating per minute. You can usually find your pulse on your wrist or carotid artery in the neck. To avoid all the bother, I strongly

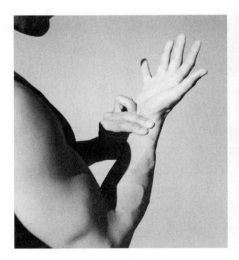 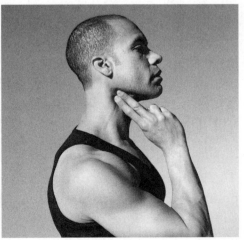

recommend investing in a heart rate monitor, a simple device that you wear on your chest or wrist. There are numerous brands of heart rate monitors on the market, including Polar, Cardiosport, and Reebok. They're all fine. In addition, many cardio machines, including exercise bikes, treadmills, and stair-climbing machines, have heart rate monitors built right into the machines.

Why not work out at 80 or 90 percent of your full potential? Pushing yourself too hard can actually hamper your fitness goals. Your body burns fat best when you are working out in the 60 to 70 percent training range. Anything beyond that may strengthen your heart but will not burn fat. Endurance athletes may benefit from a more strenuous workout, but sticking with your training goals is the best way to achieve Noble fitness. As you get more fit, your heart will become more efficient. Your resting heart rate, the number of times your heart beats per minute when you're not doing any physical activity, may go down. That's a sign that your heart is able to do more work with less effort. The average heart rate is 72 beats per minute, but well-conditioned athletes tend to have lower resting heart rates than average, sometimes as low as 50 or under. You should check your resting heart rate right when you get up in the morning, before you even get out of bed. It's easy. Just take your pulse for 10 seconds and multiply that number by 6. If an athlete's resting heart rate goes up and not down, it's a sign that he or she is overtraining and should slow down.

I outline my favorite cardio programs in this chapter, but my suggestions are by no means the final word. As long as you are working within your target heart rate, you can be creative with your cardio. You can use a standard exercise machine such as a treadmill, an exercise bike, a stair machine, or an elliptical machine if you own one or have access to one at a gym. You can also take 10-minute cardio breaks throughout the day by walking fast, running, climbing steps, running in place in front of the TV, jumping rope, skating, or dancing. The point is to get your heart pumping and your lungs working. A major side benefit of cardio is that within a short time of starting a regular cardio program, you will feel more energized and have more stamina.

how much cardio is right for you?

Lean Machine   Too much cardio can interfere with your ability to maintain muscle. You should do two to three 20- to 45-minute cardio breaks a week and don't exceed your target training zone.

Muscle Maker   You need to maintain the right balance between cardio to strengthen your heart and resistance training to keep you toned. You should do three to five 20- to 45-minute cardio breaks a week.

Fat Fighter   You need to boost your metabolism to burn off fat, and cardio is a great way to do it. You should do at least four to five 20- to 60-minute cardio breaks a week.

Refer to my Web site (www.bodynoble.com) to get a customized in-house training cardio workout and to make sure you're training at the right intensity.

the 10-minute power burst

It's best if you try to do 20 minutes of cardio at a time, but there will be days when you may only have 10 minutes at a time. When you only have 10 to spare, here's how to structure your cardio workout. Gradually warm up for the first 5 minutes. For the next 5 minutes, work at your target heart rate, and then spend a few minutes cooling down.

take the first step

We've become such an automobile-dependent society that some people barely walk at all any more. I often recommend that clients purchase a pedometer, a device you can wear on your hip that actually measures how many steps you take every day, inside your home and outdoors. The rule of thumb is that people who are considered to be at a low activity level take 2,000 steps or less daily, which is equal to walking about 1 mile.

People who are considered to be at moderate activity level take between 5,000 and 7,000 steps daily, which is equal to walking between 2½ and 3½ miles daily, and people who are in the active group take about 10,000 steps, which is equal to walking around 5 miles daily. For every 2,000 steps you take, you burn 100 calories, so if you walk the full 10,000 steps, you burn about 500 calories. Clearly, if you want to stay slim, you need to take more steps. I try to walk whenever I can. I park at the far end of a parking lot so I can get a few hundred extra steps in on my errands. I always walk up the steps if given the option. And I try to take a walk every day just to enjoy the outdoors.

power walking

Power walking—walking at a brisk pace so that you are working your cardiovascular system—is my absolute favorite exercise for several reasons. It's great for beginners because everyone knows how to walk, although there are a few simple techniques you may need to learn. Walking is beneficial for practically everyone at every age and stage in life. It is not as rough on your joints as jogging or running, yet it offers the same cardiovascular benefits. It is suitable for most people with the exception of those with severe knee, hip, or back problems. (If you have serious joint problems, swimming may be a better choice for you. And of course, you need to consult your physician before embarking on any form of exercise.) It's not boring. If you walk outdoors, you can vary your route so you see different scenery every day or so. It's portable. You can do it virtually anywhere. Best of all, it doesn't require a lot of expensive equipment. All you need is a good pair of walking or cross-training shoes (my favorite brands include New Balance, Asics, Saucony, Nike, and Adidas) and a heart rate monitor if you choose to use one. (For more information on how to buy athletic shoes, see Noble Looks on page 229.) If you prefer to work out indoors, or in the event of inclement weather, you can do your power walking program on an exercise treadmill. If given a choice, I always opt to do my cardio outdoors where I can enjoy fresh air and sunshine, and connect with nature.

Try to take a power walk three to four times a week.

I am a certified Reebok power walking specialist, which means that I have been trained to teach people the proper technique and form to pursue an effective walking program. If you've never done any form of cardio, power walking is a great way to get started.

To begin your power walking routine, be sure to get your body aligned in the correct posture. If your posture is poor—if your body is out of alignment—you will place added burden on your hips and knees, which can ultimately cause injury. Place your feet shoulder width apart with your knees slightly bent. Keep your shoulders upright and your head facing forward. Your stomach muscles should be contracted, and your arms should be bent 90 degrees with your elbows at your side. Begin your walk slowly and gradually increase your speed.

Around 10 minutes into your power walk, be sure to check whether you have reached your target heart rate. Wearing a heart rate monitor is the easiest and most practical way to keep track of whether you are working hard enough. In my experience, most people don't push themselves enough, and never reach their correct training zone. If you find that you have not yet reached your target heart rate, work harder. If you have exceeded it, lighten up.

level 1

Level 1 is for beginners. You are walking at a comfortable pace that is more than a stroll but not anywhere near a run. The correct walking form is to push off from your heel as your foot moves toward your toe. With each step, you are engaging your entire foot, not just the front or back. Keep your arms bent at a 90 degree angle and your elbows bent at your side. Move in a fluid, easy motion. If you are a beginner, try to sustain this for 30 minutes. (If you are more advanced, walk at this pace for the first 2 to 3 minutes, and then move on to Level 2.) Once Level 1 becomes easy for you, do as much of your walking program at Level 2 as you can. Eventually, you will be able to use Level 1 as a warm-up, and spend most of your time in Level 2.

level 2

Level 2 is similar to Level 1 in technique, but you will use your arms and legs to increase the intensity of your stride as you walk. Slightly shorten your strides—each step should be shorter but more powerful. This will automatically increase your leg speed. Let your arms swing naturally at your sides. Your heart rate will also increase, and you will feel that you are more actively engaging your muscles. Many people find that a half hour of walking at Level 2 intensity gives them an excellent cardio workout. If at some point you no longer feel challenged by Level 2, you can move on to Level 3. Give yourself 3 minutes to cool down before stopping. Gradually reduce your pace, and let your heart rate get back to normal.

level 3

Level 3 is a faster version of Level 2, similar to the speed-walking competitions you see at the Olympics. In Level 3, you increase your arm speed and shorten your leg stride even more. You will need to use your entire body to propel you forward. With each step, cross one foot in front of the other. This engages your hips as you move from side to side, giving you more power. Level 3 is very intense, and you may not be able to sustain it for the full 30 minutes. If you feel up to it, try to incorporate 5 or 10 minutes of Level 3 into your Level 2 workout. Give yourself 3 minutes to cool down before stopping. Gradually reduce your pace, and let your heart rate get back to normal.

after your power walk

Don't forget to do your stretches, or your muscles can get tight and sore. Stretch out your hamstrings, quadriceps, calves, and glutes. When you're done stretching, have a light post-workout snack. And don't forget to keep drinking water during your walk and throughout the day.

tips for using a treadmill or an elliptical trainer

You can do an effective power-walk program on a treadmill or an elliptical trainer, but these machines are not for everyone. You need to have reasonably good balance and coordination to use a treadmill. If you don't, hold on to the side posts for support. Be careful about mounting the treadmill, and be especially careful about getting off it. Never get off a moving treadmill—wait for the treadmill to come to a complete stop. You can alter the intensity of your workout by increasing the speed and grade of the treadmill. You can also program your training heart rate on a computerized treadmill or elliptical trainer, which makes it very easy for you to control your target heart rate.

I begin my treadmill workout with a 5-minute warm-up where I'm walking at a comfortable pace. Then I quickly pick up the pace to reach my target heart rate. Since I can get rather bored on a treadmill unless I can listen to music on my iPod, I put the treadmill on a manual setting so that I can play around with my workout. I like to switch speeds and alter the grade so I can create some variety. It makes it a lot more fun than doing the same thing all the time.

running

Running is one of my favorite cardio activities because I feel that it accomplishes a great deal in a short amount of time. Over time, a consistent running program not only strengthens your heart and lungs, it also sculpts and tones your body, especially your legs, at the same time. Running is a high-impact activity, which means it is not suitable for people with joint problems. Jogging is an easier version of running and is not quite as taxing on the body. If you have not done a running program before, jogging is a good way to begin, though jogging is not suitable for people with joint problems, either.

Before you try to jog or run, be sure to invest in a good pair of running shoes. These shoes are especially well padded in areas that must bear the most weight as you jog or run.

Whether you run or jog, you need to begin slowly. If you've never done either, I recommend starting out with my power-walking program. Once you are comfortable working at Level 3, you can begin to break into a moderate jog or run.

For both jogging and running, maintaining good posture is very important. As with power walking, your arms should be slightly bent and in at your sides. I often see recreational runners with really bad posture. They are too slouched over, which puts a lot of strain on the upper back and neck muscles.

When you jog or run, you need to do more of a warm-up than you do for power walking, or you risk injury. Before beginning your program, take 5 minutes or so to walk quickly and get the blood flowing in your legs. After you have warmed up a bit, stretch out your leg muscles, specifically your hamstrings, quadriceps, calves, and glutes. Once you're stretched out and warmed up, you can begin your program.

If you're a beginner, start off slowly and jog every other day. You need to give your joints a rest and your muscles some time to repair between jogs. Do as much as you can without getting completely exhausted. Try to work up to 25- to 30-minute sessions by adding 3 minutes per week to your jog.

If you are an advanced runner, run every other day but aim to increase your time to 3 minutes a week until you reach 45 to 60 minutes. If you need a greater challenge, add some hilly terrain to your program.

About 5 minutes into your jogging or running program, be sure to check your target heart rate. If you haven't reached it, move faster. If you have exceeded it, slow down until you bring your heart rate back down to where it should be.

Give yourself 5 minutes to cool down before you stop jogging or running. Gradually reduce your pace, letting your heart rate get back to normal.

Bring a bottle of water with you so that you stay hydrated. After

> **Noble Tip**
>
> If you are well conditioned, during your jog or run, break into a really fast run or sprint and sustain it for about a block. Then go back to your normal speed. Why? You have two different types of muscle fibers—slow-twitch fibers and fast-twitch fibers. When you walk or jog at a sustained pace, you use your slow-twitch fibers. You only use your fast-twitch fibers when you have sudden bursts of activity. Conditioning your fast-twitch fibers will help to better strengthen and tone the muscles in your legs and works your heart anaerobically.

you're finished, be sure to stretch out your hamstrings, quadriceps, calves, and glutes. Stretching will reduce post-workout discomfort and help maintain flexibility. When you're done stretching, have a light post-workout snack.

I often try to keep my clients motivated by finding a local 5k or 10k race in their community that they can train for. Many competitions raise money for worthy causes, such as research dollars for breast cancer, AIDS, or MS. By participating in these charity events, you really feel you're making a difference in people's lives. Of course, you're making a real positive difference in your own life, as well. It's great to have a specific goal to work toward, and when you make it to the finish line, you know that you've accomplished something special.

cycling

Cycling provides another terrific cardio routine you can incorporate into your weekly training program. Mixing it up keeps it from getting boring. I love riding my bike outdoors, but you can get as good a workout on a stationary bicycle at the health club or at home.

outdoor cycling

Outdoor cyclists must wear a bicycle helmet to prevent head injuries, and sunglasses or tinted goggles to protect their eyes against the sun, dust, stones, and other pieces of flying debris. Be sure to wear bicycle gloves for long rides to avoid hand blisters. People with arthritic knees may be able to ride a bicycle as long as the seat height is set correctly. Arthritic knees should not be hyperextended (bent more than 90 degrees). If your arthritis is severe, stick to a stationary bicycle as long as you cycle on it without pain.

Although it is rare, keep in mind that people do fall off bikes. In most cases, you simply brush yourself off and get back on, but there is always a risk of injury. If you have any orthopedic problems that could be made worse after even a mild fall, stick to a stationary bike.

Unlike walking, running, or jogging, cycling is not a weight-bearing activity, which means that it does not prevent osteoporosis, or the thinning of bones that makes you prone to fractures later in life. If you are also doing the Body Noble Workout, however, you are doing enough weight-bearing exercise to keep your bones strong.

For outdoor cycling, purchase a bike that suits your lifestyle. There are so many varieties to chose from, from road bikes to mountain bikes, from beach cruisers to hybrids. Go to a well-stocked bicycle shop and test out some models before you make your choice.

Aim for a 30- to 60-minute program. Thirty minutes is fine for a good cardio workout, but some people like to keep going for longer because they find it fun. Start out at a moderate pace, and work your way up to your target heart rate. When you're cycling, it's much easier to simply check your heart rate monitor than to try to measure your pulse. Try to maintain your pedal speed at 70 to 90 rpm per leg. (You don't actually count your leg rotations, a gauge on the bike does that for you!) If you can't make it to a full half-hour at first, do as much as you can without getting exhausted, and every time you go out on your bicycle, try to increase your time by 3 minutes or so. Before too long, you will have worked your way up to a half-hour. Sip water along the way as you need it.

When you're done with your bike ride, don't forget to stretch out your leg muscles, especially your glutes, hamstrings, and quads, which may feel very tight.

indoor stationary bike

An indoor stationary bike is a safe and convenient way to get a good cardio workout, and you can do it in bad weather. Just about every health club has a few stationary bikes, or you can buy one for your home. There are basically two types of bikes: upright and recumbent. Upright bikes sit higher than recumbent bikes, which are lower and are sloped downward. An upright bike gives you a better workout because you have to hold yourself up and therefore engage your core muscles as well as your leg muscles. The downside is, upright bikes are harder to use and can put pressure on your back. If you have any problems, a recumbent bike is better because you can lean back in a more comfortable position.

Many stationary bikes are computerized and can be programmed to suit your individual workout needs. When you begin your workout, input your age and weight, and the bike designs your workout for you. You can also alter the program to suit your level of fitness. You don't have to keep track of your target heart rate because the bike does it for you. If you're not working hard enough, the bike can automatically increase resistance; if you're working too hard, it can reduce resistance or slow down your speed. Some of the more expensive models have built-in monitors and places for you to pop in your favorite CD. It's not exactly a necessity, but it does make the time fly by.

If you're using a standard noncomputerized bike, you have to do the thinking yourself. Start out slowly, reach a moderate pace, and work your way up to your maximum speed by about 10 minutes into your program. Check your heart rate monitor to make sure that you have reached your target zone. Stay at your target zone for another 10 minutes, then begin to gradually cool down. When you have finished your bike ride, be sure to stretch out your muscles.

disco fit for your heart

Here's a really fun way to give your heart a good workout: Go out to a dance club. I do my best cardio on the dance floor, and it's a lot more fun than pounding the pavement running or racing up stairs. Find a club specializing in the genre of music that you really love. Is it house, salsa, ballroom, country western, techno, marengo, disco, progressive, or some other style? Plan to spend at least an hour dancing to your favorite music. Throw your heart into it. Feel your pulse pound and your heart race. Dancing is not only great cardio, it's a terrific way to relieve stress and work out your leg and abdominal muscles. Shake out the tension of the day. Be social, have fun. But don't wreck your heart-healthy experience by boozing it up or smoking. I recommend drinking mineral water and lime to keep yourself hydrated while you are active. If you drink alcohol while you're moving around, you could become dehydrated. When you've finished doing your strenuous physical activity, you can have a glass of wine or beer. My rule for booze is: Have one or have none. My rule for smoking is: No smoking. Period.

swimming

Swimming is a great cardio option, especially for people with joint problems or injuries. The buoyancy of the water reduces the stress on your joints, yet if you swim at a brisk pace, you can still give your heart and lungs a great workout. When you swim, you use all your muscle groups—your legs, your core, and your arms. Swimming strengthens and tones your body and is a great way to take off weight. The downside of swimming is that it is not a weight-bearing exercise, so it will not prevent osteoporosis. So, you need to supplement swimming with some form of resistance training.

It doesn't matter whether you swim in a pool, a lake, or even the ocean, but you need to be able to swim comfortably for about a half-hour. If cold water is not for you, look for a heated indoor pool. Always wear goggles, and if you swim outdoors, always wear waterproof sunscreen or a wet suit. If you swim in chlorinated pools on a regular basis, consider wearing a bathing cap. Chlorine can be rough on your hair, especially if it is color treated. Be sure to wash the chlorine off after the swim.

Swimming requires a lot of skill and technique, and if you're serious about starting a swimming program but aren't sure that your technique is up to par, take a few lessons before you begin. Many YM/YWCAs, health clubs, and even high schools offer swimming lessons and master swim clubs.

The most popular swimming technique is freestyle, followed by the breaststroke and the backstroke. Use any stroke you like as long as you do it well.

Always do a mild warm-up in the pool for 5 minutes before beginning your program. Swim at a comfortable pace so that your muscles get used to the water and the work.

Once you've become proficient at swimming, there are lots of ways to make your swim more challenging. I like to use pull buoys, which are flotation supports for the hips and legs that enable you to focus better on working your arms. Swimming with pull buoys warms up your midsection and upper back as you focus on improving your upper-body strength. You are also giving your heart and lungs a real run for their money. Start by doing one full length of the pool and work your way up to doing as many as you can.

If you're an advanced swimmer, find a swim club in your neighborhood that offers challenging programs. Sometimes it's fun to be spurred on by others with similar goals.

After your swim, stretch your back, neck, shoulders, and triceps. They've been working hard and deserve some attention.

rope jumping

If you only have 10 minutes to do cardio, this is a great way to do it. Jumping rope is so intense, it gives your heart and lungs a great workout in a fraction of the time normally needed. And talk about a portable exercise! Rope jumping is an excellent form of cardio because you can do it anywhere, anytime. You can pack a jump rope in your suitcase or stash one in the top drawer of your desk. And if you think rope jumping is just for kids, think again. Many boxers incorporate rope jumping into their fitness routine because it gives them a full-body workout. Rope jumping quickly tones and sculpts your body. For boxers and other high-performance athletes, rope jumping helps develop speed, agility, balance, and coordination, and it prepares your body for explosive bursts of activity. Rope jumping is not for everyone. It is a high-intensity activity that puts stress on your hips, knees, ankle joints, and feet. If you have any weakness in those areas, rope jumping is not for you. If you are overweight, check with your doctor before starting a rope jumping program. The extra weight may be putting too much pressure on your joints.

There are numerous types of jump ropes on the market, from old-fashioned cloth ropes to leather to high-tech nylon. Choose whichever rope you like.

Rope jumping can put a lot of wear and tear on your feet. Be sure to wear a pair of cross-training shoes with ample padding in the front, because rope jumping requires bouncing and balancing your body weight on the balls of your feet. This is just the opposite of running shoes, which provide padding underneath the heels.

Don't try to jump rope on a slippery surface or a hard floor. Place a rubber mat on concrete, tile, or other hard surfaces. A wood floor is fine because it has some give to it.

You don't need to learn a lot of fancy footwork, but there are two basic steps that you need to know to get the most out of a rope jumping routine: the Basic Bounce Step and the Alternate Foot Step.

Basic Bounce Step   This is a no-brainer. Jump up and down with both feet together. At first, you may miss a few steps if you're out of practice, but within a short time, you should be able to jump without stopping.

Alternate Foot Step   Swing the rope around and jump over it with one foot at a time. Continue alternating your feet, lifting your knees slightly as if you are jogging in place. Don't kick your feet back or they may catch on the rope.

Beginners should practice these two techniques for 5 minutes, for 2 to 3 times a week until they are completely comfortable with jumping rope. Competitive athletes should practice these techniques for 10 to 15 minutes, for 3 to 5 times per week. Remember, the focus is on the skill.

It's best to divide your jump rope routine into 5 minute intervals, with 30 second rests in between. Do a 5 minute warm-up at a comfortable but brisk pace, then slow down for about 30 seconds to restore your energy, then move up the intensity for the next 5 minutes, keeping an eye on your target heart rate. Slow down for 30 seconds of rest, then finish up at a comfortable pace, but still feeling like you're working. Believe me, it's quite a workout.

After each rope jumping session, stretch out your leg muscles. They've been working hard and need to loosen up.

stair climbing

Want a pair of shapely legs? Stair climbing is the way to get them. All you need is a pair of cross-training shoes and some steps.

You can climb stairs in your office or apartment building as long as it is well lit and safe, or you can use the stair-climber machine at the gym. If you choose to use real stairs, be sure to warm up for 5 minutes by walking rapidly on flat terrain. This will get the blood flowing to your muscles before you begin your climb. It is absolutely essential to maintain good posture while climbing stairs. If you don't, you can put excess strain on your back and knee joints. Keep your spine in a neutral position with your abdominals contracted and your neck and head held upright looking straight ahead. Position your knees over your ankles to prevent strain on your knees. That way, your feet and ankles absorb some of the stress that would have burdened your knees. Focus on stepping with the ball of your foot on the step and feel the muscles contract in the back of your legs, quadriceps, and gluteal muscles. If you're starting out, try to get through a few flights at one time before quitting. Try to keep going for about 10 minutes if you can, then cool down for 5 minutes on flat ground. Check your heart rate after the first 5 minutes of climbing to make sure that you are working within your target heart rate. (Needless to say, be sure to do stair climbing in well-lit, safe areas. I also recommend that women do their stair climbing with a friend.)

The same basic rules apply if you use a stair machine at the gym. The machine will start you off with a brief warm-up and end with a cool-down. Be vigilant about maintaining good posture and not letting your knees go past your ankles. Remember to check your heart rate about 5 minutes into the workout to make sure that you are at your correct training level. Some stair machines are computerized, so that once you enter your age, weight, and desired level of workout intensity, the machine designs a program that works you at your target heart rate.

9

commonly asked questions about working out

Through the years, I've trained hundreds of clients, and have been asked countless questions about working out. Here I will answer some of the questions that I am most frequently asked about fitness.

I've just begun the Body Noble Program. How soon will I begin to see results?

Starting a fitness program is like planting a new seed in the ground: If you nurture the seed, if you water it and make sure it's exposed to sun, it will begin to sprout new roots. You may not see any concrete evidence of growth for a few weeks, but one day you'll wake up and find a new plant. The same is true about embarking on a muscle-toning and cardio regimen. You may not *see* overnight results, but within two weeks or so, you should begin to *feel* palpably better. If you eat well, get enough rest, and are consistent about working out, you will notice that you're getting stronger and more flexible. You'll probably have more energy, and may find that you're sleeping better and experiencing some of the other side benefits of following a regular workout program. Within a month or so, you will begin to see real benefits, such as a smaller waist size, more toned muscles, and less body fat. If you keep going, it will just get better and better.

Should I eat before I work out, or after?

The answer is both—you need to eat before you work out and when you're done. Before working out, you should eat something light that will give your cells fuel for energy but won't weigh you down. It's no fun doing abdominal work with a full stomach! I recommend eating a piece of fruit or half of a protein bar about 30 minutes before starting your workout. (My favorite protein bars are Organic Food Bar and Tri-O-Plex.) You should also have a snack within 10 minutes post-workout to restore the carbohydrate and protein burned by your cells for energy. Good choices include a protein shake with fresh fruit made from whey protein, a piece of fruit, and some low-fat cheese or half a protein bar. Don't forget to drink lots of water before, during, and after your workout.

My friend, who's a real gym rat, says it's not possible to get a good workout without lifting weights or using exercise machines. Am I really getting as good a workout with the exercise ball and cable?

You may be surprised to learn that in my opinion, you're getting a better workout using an exercise ball and cable than you would using fancy gym equipment. Exercise machines are designed to isolate a particular muscle group. As you move along the circuit, you go from machine to machine, each one working a specific body part. On most machines, you're sitting down. In a sense, much of the work is being done for you. Sure, you still have to move the weight on the machine to work the muscle, but it's a lot easier than having to maintain your posture while you do your exercise standing up or trying not to fall off the exercise ball. In contrast, when you're using a ball and cable, you are forced to engage more than one set of muscles at a time. You may not realize it, but "non-working" muscles in your body are actually actively helping to maintain your balance. Furthermore, I believe that once you learn the Noble

Technique, you won't need a machine to isolate your muscles for you—you will be able to do that for yourself. When you isolate and focus on each muscle group as you work it, you are improving your overall coordination because you're training your brain as well as your body. You're also training your body to be a better multitasker. Think about it. How many times does your body just do one thing? Even when you're walking, you may be carrying a bag of groceries or reaching for something overhead. You need good communication between your brain and your muscles to carry on life's activities, especially as you get older. So use your exercise ball and cable, and be proud of it. As far as lifting weights, I challenge your friend to work with a high-resistance exercise cable. It's just as hard.

Is it okay to work out when I'm tired?

As I tell my clients, it's important to listen to your body. If your body is saying, "I'm exhausted," don't try to do a strenuous workout. You probably won't get much out of it anyway. The real question is, why are you exhausted? Are you getting enough sleep at night? Be sure to get between 7 and 9 hours of sleep so that you have the physical stamina to do your workout. Are you skipping meals, so that your blood sugar is sagging? Proper nutrition is essential for providing the fuel for your workout, so be sure to eat your three meals and two snacks a day as directed in Noble Nutrition in chapter 13. Are you partying too much at night? Excess alcohol can sap your body of important nutrients such as B vitamins, which can leave you very, very tired. When it comes to drinking, stick to my rule: *One or none!*

Even if you feel like you're running on empty, you may still be able to engage in light activity, or as I call it, active rest. A nice leisurely walk in the park, a relaxing in-line skate, or a short bike ride might help reinvigorate your tired body. Even some mild stretching and breathing exercises may help you feel better. But if you're really tired, don't push yourself. Put your workout off for another day.

Should I work out if I'm coming down with a cold, or already have one?

Definitely not. When you're under the weather, you need to conserve your energy so you can get better. When your body is battling a cold or other infection, it's telling you to rest and take it easy. When I have a cold, I pamper myself. I get a large container of my favorite Asian-style chicken soup from my local Thai restaurant, drink lots of fluid (especially green tea and honey), put on my favorite CD, and read a book or nap. I use a product called Emer-gen-C, a drink mix that contains 1,000 mg of vitamin C plus other vitamins and minerals. I also suck on a zinc lozenge to soothe my throat, which helps speed recovery. I have found the herb echinacea to be helpful if I take it at the first sign of an infection. It seems to shorten the duration of a cold or flu. When I begin to feel better, I gradually return to my fitness routine. I begin by doing a light-resistance workout (I stick to an intensity level of about 3 on the Noble Rating Scale) and take a slow-paced walk in the fresh air. Within a few days, I'm roaring back to life and ready for a new challenge.

I've been working out for a few months but feel like I've stopped making any progress. Is this normal?

By not making progress I assume you mean that you don't feel that you're getting stronger and/or don't see any improvement in your body. This is a very common complaint among weight lifters and serious athletes and just about anyone who works out consistently. Here are some factors that could be causing your problem. Are you doing the same workout day after day? If you don't mix it up a bit, that is, do different exercises every few workouts, your muscles becomes accustomed to the workout and no longer find it challenging. That's why I sometimes offer a choice of two exercises for the same muscle group and suggest that you alternate between them daily or weekly. I also think that people become complacent after they have been doing the same exercises day after day, week after week. Are you still focusing on squeezing your muscles? Are you still working at the correct level of resistance or are you simply rushing through your workout without giving it all you've got? Review the

Body Noble Rating Scale on page 25, and make sure that you are working each muscle to your appropriate level of intensity. If the Body Noble Basic Workout is beginning to feel stale to you, I recommend that you try the On-the-Go workout (chapter 10) for a week or two to get your juices flowing again and then go back to the Basic Workout. Or do a combination of the Basic Workout and the On-the-Go workout. You will feel reinvigorated by the experience, and I promise you will begin to make progress once again.

I've always been active, and now that I'm in my first trimester of pregnancy, I want to continue working out for as long as I can. What kinds of exercises should I do, and which ones should I avoid?

Some of my favorite clients have been women who are eager to stay fit throughout pregnancy so that they can have a healthy baby and an easier delivery and recovery. These women are extremely motivated to take care of themselves and tend to go the extra mile to stay strong and well. First and foremost, consult with your obstetrician before you embark on any exercise program during pregnancy because there are medical conditions that may not respond well to exercise and may put the fetus at risk.

The vast majority of pregnant women, however, will benefit from regular exercise. In fact, the American College of Obstetricians and Gynecologists recommends that all healthy pregnant women exercise for about 30 minutes a day. Regular exercise during pregnancy offers numerous benefits, including reduced back pain, less undesirable weight gain, an easier labor and delivery, and an easier time getting back to normal weight after delivery.

When I work with pregnant clients, my goal is to help them maintain their strength and flexibility without exhausting them or putting their pregnancy at risk. I don't think that pregnant women should lift heavy weights, do high-impact exercises like jumping or step class, or do exercises on their back, which can put pressure on the uterus. During pregnancy, women tend to overheat quickly, so they must be careful about not exercising in hot or humid environments. Before every workout, it's a good idea to eat a small snack to avoid sudden drops in blood sugar. And of course, it's essential to keep the body cool and hydrated during exercise by drinking lots of water.

Often, women are very tired during the first trimester, and I don't want them to push themselves to a state of exhaustion. I recommend rest if they need it. By the second trimester, women usually find that they have more energy and stamina and may be able to exercise for longer periods of time. I don't have a specific exercise regimen for pregnancy, but I do modify my existing program. I typically start pregnant women off with a power walking cardio program at a moderate pace so that they can get a good workout without overheating their bodies. While normal-weight women should gain between 25 and 35 pounds during pregnancy, many women gain way too much weight and have a really rough time taking it off later. Cardio helps to prevent unwanted weight gain during pregnancy, and it is great for overall fitness. It's good to incorporate light resistance exercises into a basic training program. You can do most of the Body Noble Workout as long as you avoid doing exercises on your back, or any exercise that makes you feel unstable. If you don't feel secure on the exercise ball, especially late in your pregnancy, don't do the exercise. And don't work to your max—work at around Levels 2 or 3, but no higher! You can also do some mild stretching, *mild* being the operative word. Pregnancy hormones can make your joints more flexible, and therefore weaker and more injury-prone. Take extra time to warm up before working out and to cool down after working out. Begin each activity at a slow pace and gradually work your way up to your desired goal. Cool down just as slowly and carefully. It's important to avoid sudden changes in blood pressure, which can make you feel faint. Swimming and aqua fitness classes are terrific low-impact exercises that are tailor-made for pregnancy. They work every muscle in the body, and the buoyancy of water will make you feel less burdened by all the added weight. They're also soothing to your joints.

At what point should you stop exercising? Some women continue doing mild exercise practically right up to delivery, others may need to stop earlier. This is a judgment call that should be made by your doctor.

Most women should be able to resume exercise about six weeks after delivery. Start slowly and give yourself a few weeks to work yourself back into your normal exercise regimen.

One final caveat: If you have problems during exercise, feel faint, or experience any unusual symptoms, call your physician.

My muscles ache the day after I work out. Am I working out too hard?

It's reasonable to experience some mild muscle or joint soreness after a workout. Remember, you make muscle by creating microscopic tears in muscle fiber, which will ultimately make muscles grow bigger but in the process may produce some inflammation. Post-workout discomfort should be relatively mild and not painful. Try putting an ice pack on an overworked muscle or joint for about 10 minutes every few hours. This should relieve the discomfort. You definitely should not be working out to the point that you are in pain the next day. That's a sign that you are overdoing it and should scale back the intensity of your workout. Bathing in Epsom salts can help alleviate post-workout soreness.

I sometimes wake up with an ache in my lower back. Can I still work out?

Anytime someone tells me they're in pain, I take it seriously. If you have a chronic pain in your lower back—or anywhere else—you should have it checked out by your doctor. It could just be a sign of weak back muscles or it could be a symptom of another problem. Once you've excluded another medical problem, focus on why you're in pain. In most cases, a sore back (or a sore knee, or an aching ankle) is due to a weakness somewhere in your body that is throwing off your alignment and making you prone to injury. A mild strength-training program designed by a qualified physical therapist is the best way for you to proceed with your exercise routine. Once the problem is healed, you can probably go back to your usual workout.

I believe in listening to your body. Pain is a sign of inflammation and swelling in your muscles, joints, tendons, or ligaments. Working when you're in pain will only make it worse. I recommend the standard RICE therapy, an acronym for Rest, Ice, Compression, and Elevation. Rest the area in pain for 48 hours. Ice it down every 10 to 15 minutes. Compress the area by wrapping an elastic bandage (such as an ACE bandage) around the injury if it makes it feel better. And try to keep the injured area elevated if possible. Once the pain subsides, you can resume your normal workout routine. I explain more about the care of injuries in chapter 14, Strengthening Your Weak Links.

I used to be very active and worked out a few times a week and regularly did cardio. After hitting a really busy time at work a few months ago, I stopped exercising altogether. Now I'm having difficulty resuming an exercise routine. Any advice on how to get motivated and how to get myself back into a program?

Your situation is not unusual for someone with a busy life. The constant tug-of-war between work, kids, family obligations, or illness can make it difficult to fit fitness into our lives. Unfortunately, the very thing that gives you the stamina and energy to get through the day—your exercise program—is often the first to go! How do you get started again? First, I think you need to understand that fitness is not a luxury, it's a necessity. You are putting your mental and physical health at risk if you don't do some form of exercise on a regular basis. You will be able to perform better on the job and at home if you are working out. I suggest that you read the introduction again for further inspiration.

The most important first step is to take that first step. And I mean this literally. Get moving! Start getting back into cardio by doing one of my fun cardio programs. Power walking is a good way to begin because you don't have to learn any special skills. Make a promise to yourself that you'll take a 20-minute walk every other day, weather permitting. If it's raining or cold, you can walk at an indoor mall or gym, or you can just dance for 20 minutes at home to your favorite music. Don't make a big deal about resuming your resistance training. The more obstacles you build up in your head, the harder it will be. Getting started is easier than you think. Grab your exercise ball and exercise cable and begin doing a few of the exercises that appeal to you in the Body Noble Workout.

Go slowly at first. Ease yourself into the program. Make it fun: Put on your iPod. Give yourself a few days to learn the exercises, then write out a schedule for yourself. When is the best time of day for you to exercise? Can you do some of your workout at the office? Please review my Body Noble On-the-Go Workout on page 125. Given your work life, it may make sense for you to do the Body Noble Basic Workout at home on the weekends, and the On-the-Go Workout during the week during some down time at the office. Once you get going, within a short time you're going to feel so much better that you're going to wonder why you ever stopped.

10

body noble
on-the-go workout

Are you spending more time at work or at school these days than you do at home? These basic exercises and stretches can be done anywhere you have access to a chair, a table, and a few feet of floor space. This is a great workout for the office, but you can also do it at home on days that you don't have access to any exercise equipment, or just want a change. In chapter 11, Body Noble Lifestyle Fitness, I show you how to modify this program so you can stay fit in more exotic locales, including hotel rooms, and airport terminals—and even the front seat of your car.

Before you do an On-the-Go exercise, take a few seconds to review the Noble Technique. Get a mental image of the muscle you are working and remember what it *feels* like when that muscle is fully engaged. Actually touch the muscle before you do the exercise. The extra few seconds of preparation will result in a better, more effective workout.

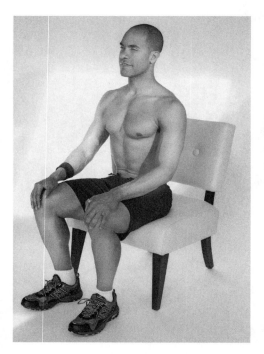

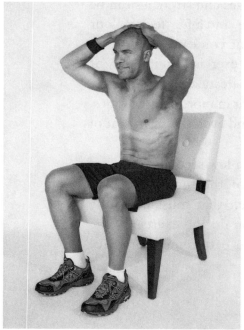

Seated Abdominal Crunch

This exercise takes the tension off your lower back as well as strengthening and toning your midsection. It's a great exercise to do at the office.

Equipment needed: Chair

Working muscles: Abs

1. Sit up tall in a straight-back chair and imagine that you have a water balloon in your abdominal area that you need to squeeze. Lace your fingers together behind your head and keep your chin up.

2. Lean over slightly as you contract your abdominal muscles. The action is similar to the ab crunch machine at the gym, but you can create your own resistance by maintaining the squeeze. Hold the squeeze for 5 seconds.

Lean Machine   Do two sets, 15 to 20 repetitions per set.

Muscle Maker   Do two sets, 15 to 20 repetitions per set.

Fat Fighter   Do two sets, 15 to 20 repetitions per set.

Seated Reverse Crunch

Equipment needed: Chair

Working muscles: Lower abs

1. Sit up tall in a straight-backed chair with your feet flat on the ground. Don't slouch! Place your hands at the side of your seat for support.

2. Contract your abdominal muscles and pick your feet up off the floor. Hold the squeeze for 5 seconds. Use your ab muscles to lift your legs and hold the squeeze for 2 seconds. With control, bring your feet back to the floor and don't rely on momentum.

3. Return to the starting position.

Lean Machine   Do two sets, 15 to 20 repetitions per set.

Muscle Maker   Do two sets, 15 to 20 repetitions per set.

Fat Fighter   Do two sets, 15 to 20 repetitions per set.

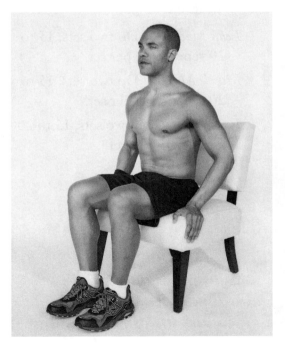 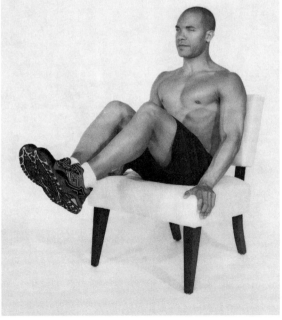

Elevated Leg Crunch

Equipment needed: Chair, bed, or sofa
Working muscles: Abs

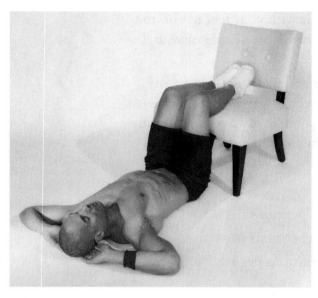

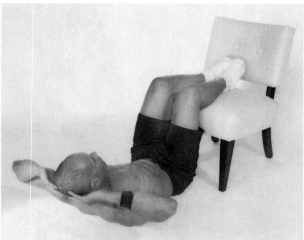

1. Lie flat on your back on the floor with your feet raised on a chair, bed, or sofa.

2. Suck in your breath and draw your navel toward your spine. Inhale deeply, then slowly lift your shoulders as you crunch toward your knees and away from the floor. Imagine that there is a tennis ball under your chin to keep your head in alignment.

3. Pause and return to the starting position.

Lean Machine Do two sets, 15 to 20 repetitions per set.

Muscle Maker Do two sets, 15 to 20 repetitions per set.

Fat Fighter Do two sets, 15 to 20 repetitions per set.

Bicycle Crunch

Equipment needed: Towel or mat

Working muscles: Obliques (side abs)

1. Lie flat on your back on a towel or mat with your knees bent at 90 degrees so that they are directly above your hips.

2. Gently support your head with your finger tips and point your elbows out to the sides.

3. Inhale, and bring your navel in toward your spine.

4. Exhale as you slowly draw your left knee toward your chest and right shoulder toward your knee, keeping your lower back lightly in contact with the floor. Pause, then switch your legs and bring your right knee toward your chest and left shoulder. Repeat the exercise to complete 1 repetition. This exercise should feel like riding a bicycle while lying on your back.

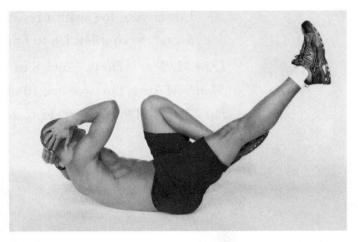

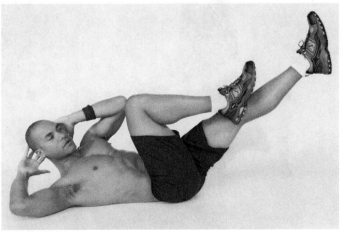

Lean Machine   Do two sets, 15 to 20 repetitions per set.

Muscle Maker   Do two sets, 15 to 20 repetitions per set.

Fat Fighter   Do two sets, 15 to 20 repetitions per set.

Seated Leg Extension

Equipment needed: Chair

Working muscles: Quads

1. Sit up tall in a straight-backed chair.

2. Extend your right leg straight out in front of you. Imagine that your leg is in a big bowl of quicksand as you contract your left quadricep (thigh) muscles. Work hard! Try to focus on the squeeze as you straighten your knee. Hold for 2 seconds. Squeeze it!

3. Lower your leg against resistance.

4. Switch to your left leg to finish one complete set.

Lean Machine   Do two sets, 8 to 10 repetitions per set.

Muscle Maker   Do two sets, 10 to 15 repetitions per set.

Fat Fighter   Do two sets, 15 to 20 repetitions per set.

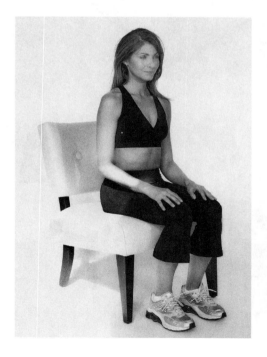 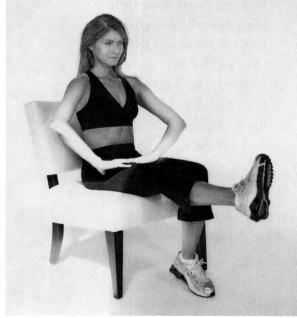

Seated Calf Raise

If you want shapely legs, this is an exercise for you.

Equipment needed: Chair optional

Working muscles: Calves

1. Place your feet shoulder width apart and sit with your body in neutral alignment.

2. While seated, slowly raise your lower leg up onto the tips of your toes and dip your heels back down toward the floor. You will really feel the burn in your calf muscles.

Lean Machine   Do two sets, 8 to 10 repetitions per set.

Muscle Maker   Do two sets, 10 to 15 repetitions per set.

Fat Fighter   Do two sets, 15 to 20 repetitions per set.

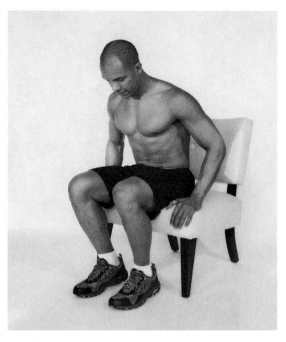

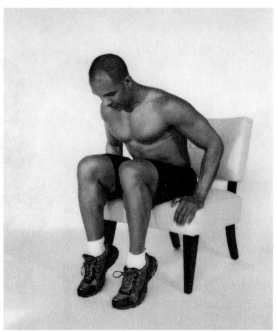

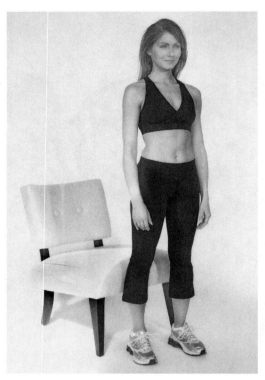

Chair Butt Squat

Equipment needed: Chair or sofa

Working muscles: Glutes

1. Stand up straight in front of a chair or sofa with your body in neutral alignment and your feet shoulder width apart.

2. With your arms extended in front of you for balance, bend your knees and sit back into a squatting position into a chair, but don't actually sit down. Try to stop before your butt touches the seat.

3. Stand up and repeat the exercise. Feel the contraction in your butt and thigh muscles. This will help strengthen and sculpt your lower body.

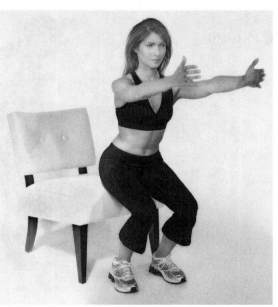

Lean Machine   Do two sets, 8 to 10 repetitions per set.

Muscle Maker   Do two sets, 10 to 15 repetitions per set.

Fat Fighter   Do two sets, 15 to 20 repetitions per set.

Lunges

Lunges are the fastest way to tone your butt and lower body. This is also a great exercise to do if you've been sitting for a while and feel stiff. Avoid lunges if you have knee problems.

Equipment needed: Chair

Working muscles: Glutes, hamstrings, and quads

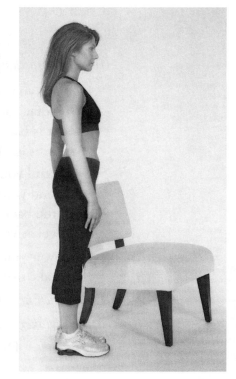

1. Stand up tall at the side of a stable chair in neutral alignment with your feet shoulder width apart. Place your left hand on the chair for support.

2. Step forward with your right leg and place your right foot on the floor in front of you. As you step forward, your back leg will bend from the knee, but should not touch the floor. Push back and feel the squeeze in your left leg and butt muscles. Stay in control. Be sure not to let your knees extend over your toes. Don't lean on the chair, merely use it to stabilize you. Do the work with your leg muscles, not your arm muscles.

3. Do one full set of lunges on one leg, then switch to the other to complete the set.

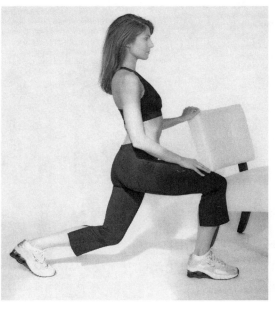

Lean Machine   Do two sets, 8 to 10 repetitions per set.

Muscle Maker   Do two sets, 10 to 15 repetitions per set.

Fat Fighter   Do two sets, 15 to 20 repetitions per set.

Chair Dip

Equipment needed: Chair or sofa

Working muscles: Triceps and shoulders

1. Place your hands shoulder width apart on the edge of a chair or sofa. Your feet should also be shoulder width apart. Your butt is barely touching the edge of the chair and your body weight is supported by your arms.

2. Extend your elbows 90 degrees and raise your body as you extend your elbows. Don't lock your elbows. Feel the squeeze in the back of your arms. Imagine that you are wringing out a towel as you lift up your body.

3. Lower yourself back down carefully. Don't allow momentum to take over. Stay in control.

Lean Machine   Do two sets, 8 to 10 repetitions per set.

Muscle Maker   Do two sets, 10 to 15 repetitions per set.

Fat Fighter   Do two sets, 15 to 20 repetitions per set.

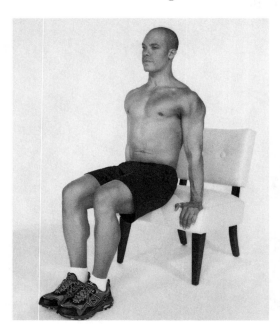 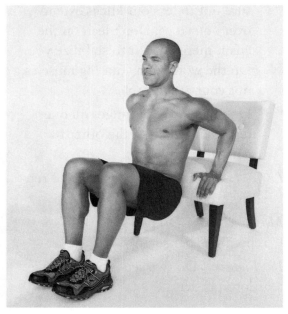

Neck Stretch

After you've been sitting at your desk staring at a computer screen or holding the phone to your ear for hours, this is a great exercise to relieve the stress in your neck.

Equipment needed: Chair optional

Working muscles: Neck and upper back

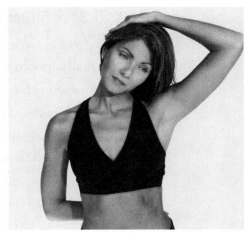

1. In a standing or seated position, flex your neck to your left side and feel the stretch in your side neck muscles. Use your left hand to gently assist the stretch. Don't yank at your neck. Hold for 10 seconds.

2. Flex your neck to the right side. Use your right hand to gently assist the stretch. Hold for 10 seconds.

3. Flex your neck straight down toward your chest. Use both hands to gently assist the stretch. Hold for 10 seconds.

4. Flex your neck down but on an angle to your left side. Use your left hand to gently assist the stretch. Hold for 10 seconds.

5. Flex your neck down but on an angle to your right side. Use your right hand to gently assist the stretch. Hold for 10 seconds.

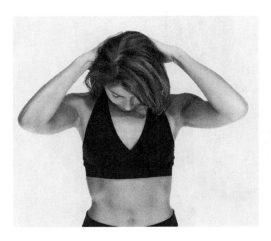

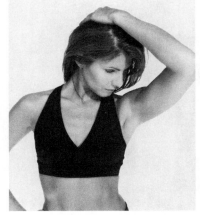

Mid-Back Stretches

I do these exercises all day long, sitting or standing. They feel great and really loosen up those tight back muscles.

Equipment needed: Chair

Working muscles: Mid-back and neck

1. Sit in a chair and clasp your hands with your arms fully extended in front of you.

2. As you bend over at your waist, place your hands under your knees and pull your elbows toward your feet.

3. Feel the stretch in your mid-back as you attempt to pull on your hands.

4. Hold the stretch for 10 seconds and exhale.

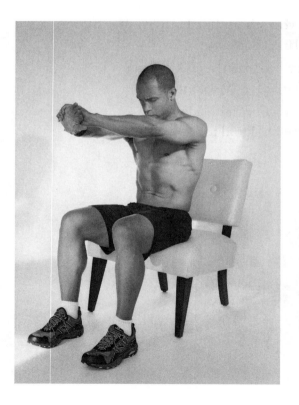 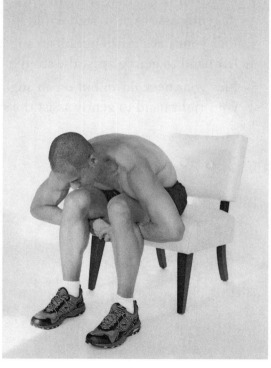

Lower-Back Stretch

Equipment needed: Chair

Working muscles: Lower back and spine

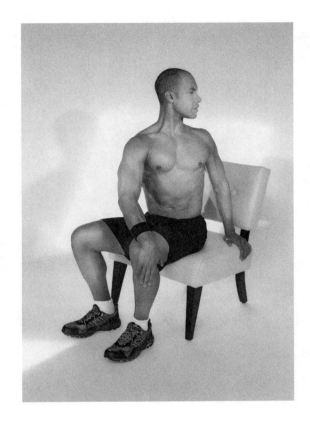

1. Sit up tall in a straight-backed chair. Rotate your body so that your right arm rests on the outside of your right thigh.

2. Place your left arm on the left side of the chair as you rotate and stretch the muscles around your spine and lower back from the waist. You will feel this in your spinal muscles and lower back. Hold for 10 seconds. Exhale during the stretch.

3. Repeat on the other side and hold each side for 10 seconds. Exhale during the stretch.

Push-Up

See photos and directions on page 67.

body noble lifestyle fitness

So you think there's no time to work out? Not true! Whether you're at work, doing housework, commuting, on the road, or vegging out in front of the TV, you can *squeeze* (pun intended) in a few exercises and stretches. Here are some easy ways to incorporate Body Noble On-the-Go exercises into your everyday life.

the office pump

You may have a desk job, but it doesn't mean that you have to be sedentary. Here are four simple exercises you can do right at your desk that will help strengthen and tone your lower body and improve blood flow to your legs. These exercises will help prevent that stiff, achy feeling you can get after sitting for hours on end with no activity.

Seated Abdominal Crunch

All you need is a chair and a few quiet minutes to yourself. If you don't have time to do your abs when you do your Body Noble Workout, you can do them at your desk.

See photos and directions on page 126.

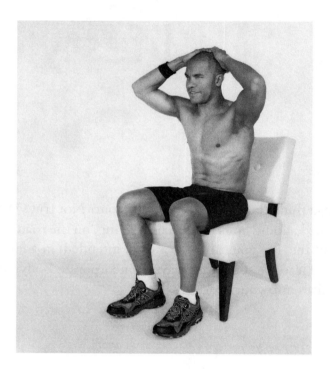

Seated Leg Extension

See photos and directions on page 130.

Seated Calf Raise

See photos and directions on page 131.

Chair Butt Squat

When you sit all day on your butt, your muscles can become untoned. This exercise is a great way to lift and tighten up your butt. When you have a break at work, you can walk over to the vending machine and get some cookies or chips—or you can use the time to make yourself look better in or out of your clothes. The choice is yours! See photos and directions on page 132.

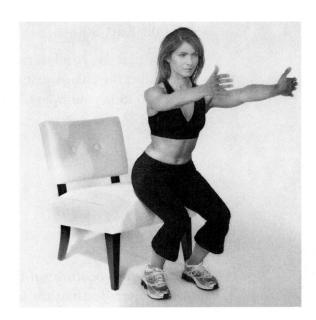

jet set fitness workout

Do you sometimes feel as if you are living out of your suitcase? I know the feeling. I travel a lot for business and I understand that staying fit on the road can be a challenge. Fortunately, many hotels now have excellent fitness facilities, but even so, you may not have time to take advantage of the hotel gym. Here are some easy ways to stay fit on the road.

Airport Terminal Walk

You breezed through airport security—now you have some time to kill at the airport. You can put it to good use. Give yourself a brisk walk around the terminal. You don't have to break into a full sweat to get the physical and mental benefits of a leisure walk program; all you need to do is to get your heart pumping a bit faster than normal. Be sure to check your flight departure time before you begin your walk—I don't want you to miss your plane. And don't forget to buy a big bottle of water to keep you well hydrated on the flight.

Chair Butt Squat

Now that you're all warmed up from your walk, you can do that old standby, the chair squat, in a quiet part of the terminal. It's a great way to tone your upper legs and butt. See photos and directions on page 132.

On-board Fitness

Maintain good posture on the plane while you are sitting or you'll arrive at your destination with a neck- or backache. Place a small pillow behind you to support your lower back. This helps to keep your back in a neutral position. I also recommend using a cervical or circular-shaped pillow for long flights to support your neck. Always be sure that you are in a comfortable position for the flight. I know that on some flights leg room is scarce, so it is critical that you get up and walk around as much as possible to keep the blood circulating properly throughout your body and to prevent blood clots. Go to a quiet part of the plane (usually the back) and do these easy stretches and exercises.

Overhead Arm Stretch

1. Put your hands over your head and try to reach up toward the roof of the plane.
2. Hold the stretch for 10 seconds. You should feel this in your arms and back. Repeat 10 times.

Bend-Over Stretch

1. Place your feet shoulder width apart and bend over at your waist. Keep your legs loose and don't lock your knees.
2. Hold the stretch for 15 seconds. You should feel this stretch in your lower back muscles and hamstrings.

Toe Raise

1. Place your feet shoulder width apart. Lift yourself until you are standing on the tips of your toes.
2. Drop your heels back down toward the floor. You should feel this in your calf muscles.
3. Repeat 10 times.

Go back to your seat and finish up with the following three stretches.

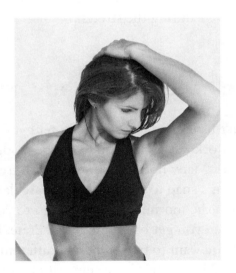

Seated Neck Stretch

Long plane rides can give anyone a stiff neck. These neck exercises can keep your neck relaxed and flexible. See photos and directions on page 135.

Seated Mid-Back Stretch

1. Place your seat in its upright position. Bend over in your seat and place your hands under your legs.
2. Grasp your hands together and point your elbows out toward the seat in front of you. Feel the stretch in your mid-back as you attempt to pull on your hands.
3. Hold the stretch for 10 seconds and exhale.

Seated Lower-Back Stretch

1. Sit up tall in your seat. Rotate your body so that your left arm rests on the right side of your right thigh.
2. Place your right arm on the right side as you rotate and stretch the muscles around your spine and lower back from the waist. You will feel this in your spinal muscles and lower back. Hold for 10 seconds. Exhale during the stretch.
3. Repeat on the other side and hold for 10 seconds. Exhale during the stretch.

the hotel room body noble pump

Don't have time to visit the hotel gym? Get yourself pumped with this easy workout. When you're on the road, don't forget to take your cardio breaks. Many hotels have gyms with treadmills or exercise bicycles that make it a snap to get your cardiovascular workout. All it takes is 10 minutes in the morning before you go to your meetings, and another 10 or so when you get back, and it's all done. If the cardio machines are taken or if you want to try something different, you can do what I do: Take the stairs. Most hotels have staircases that are rarely used. I get up early in the morning, put on my iPod, and quickly walk the steps. (Of course, only do this in safe, well-lit areas!) If you want to try this, be sure to focus on getting your full foot on the step. Squeeze your butt and leg muscles from step to step and you will work your lower body as well as your heart. If you are more advanced, you can try running the steps. Run in a straight line to the top, but when you descend the steps, don't go straight down. Descend with an S-curve motion, which takes some of the pressure off your knees. Before beginning your stair workout, be sure that the stairwell is safe and well lit.

If you don't want to run the steps, you can run in place for 10 minutes in your hotel room in front of the TV, jump rope, or do old fashioned jumping jacks as long as you don't have any knee problems.

Once you've warmed up, you can begin the Hotel Room Circuit Pump-Up. In about 10 minutes, you can work most of your major muscle groups.

Push-Up

Push-ups are a great anywhere, anytime exercise.
See photos and directions on page 67.

Standard Abdominal Crunch

See photos and directions on page 60.

Oblique Crunch (*Left Side-Right Side*)

See photos and directions on page 63.
Repeat this circuit routine three times, get into the shower, towel off, and you're ready for that important meeting.

the traffic jam pump

Feel as if you live in your car? Here is a streamlined upper-body workout that you can do when you are stuck in a traffic jam (which happens a lot in most urban areas), or after you have reached your destination, and want to do a quick exercise before you go to work or go shopping. Needless to say, don't do these exercises when you are driving—do them only when your car is at a complete stop and the gear set in park.

Steering Wheel Squeeze

1. Shift your car into park. Don't do this exercise if your car is moving!
2. Sit up tall in your car and place your hands on opposite sides of the steering wheel at the 9 o'clock and 3 o'clock positions.
3. Squeeze the steering wheel together from both sides. Feel the squeeze in your arms and chest muscles. Hold the squeeze for 5 seconds. Repeat 5 times.
4. Now slide one hand to the bottom of the steering wheel, the 6 o'clock position, and the other to the top, the 12 o'clock

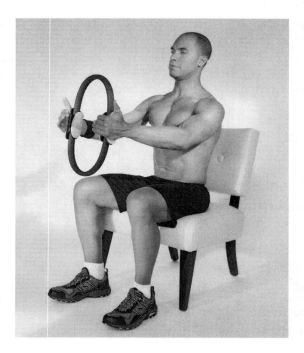
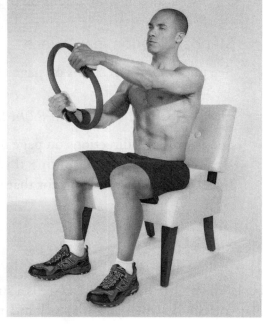

position. Squeeze both hands and feel the squeeze in your biceps. Hold for 5 seconds and repeat 5 times.

5. Now slide one hand to the 10 o'clock position on the steering wheel, and the other to the 5 o'clock position. Squeeze the steering wheel on both sides. Feel the squeeze in your shoulders. Hold for 5 seconds and repeat 5 times.

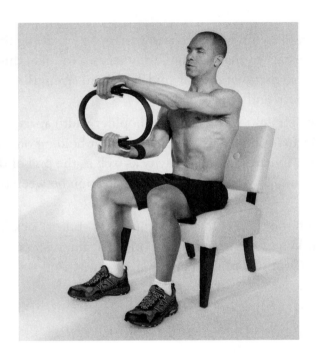

Abdominal Squeeze

1. Shift your car into park.
2. Sit back in your car seat and focus on squeezing your abdominal muscles as you slightly bend forward while contracting your abs.
3. Hold the ab squeeze for 5 seconds. Repeat 5 times.

the commuter pump

Here are some fun exercises you can do on the train, subway, or bus during your commute to work. They really work!

Train Stop Leg Pump

No one on the train will even know that you are doing this exercise unless you start to make some funny faces. No joke, this is a great core exercise that works your mid-body and strengthens and tones your abs, butt, and upper legs.

1. Sit up straight with your feet shoulder width apart. Raise your body just 1 inch above the seat without holding on to anything. You are resisting gravity as well as the pull of the moving train. Try to maintain this leg position between train stops.

2. When the train comes to a stop, relax and sit back in your seat. When the train starts to move again, resume the exercise. Continue to do this exercise between stops for 5 to 10 stops.

Seated Abdominal Crunch

1. Sit up tall in your seat and imagine that you have a water balloon in your abdominal area.

2. Lean over slightly as you contract your abdominal muscles. The action is similar to the ab crunch machine at the gym, but you have to create your own resistance by maintaining the squeeze. Hold the squeeze for 5 seconds. Do between 12 and 15 repetitions. (If you have time, do two sets. Just don't miss your stop!)

Toe Raise

Can't get a seat? While you're standing, you can work your calf muscles.

1. Place your feet shoulder width apart. Lift yourself up to the tip of your toes.
2. Drop your heels back down toward the floor. You should feel this in your calf muscles.
3. Repeat 10 times.

Stair Leg Pump

Don't think of it as an annoying flight of steps, think of it as a free lower-body workout. Stairs can be a blessing if you use them to your advantage. Don't take the elevator but walk the stairs at the bus or train station. For maximum benefit, try to get your full foot on the step and push off toward the next step. If you are very fit, take two steps at a time. Focus on squeezing your butt and leg muscles on each step.

the couch potato workout

Here's an easy, effective workout you can do right in front of your TV.

Couch Squat

This exercise tones your glutes and upper legs.

1. Stand up straight in front of your couch with your body in neutral alignment and your feet shoulder width apart.
2. Bend your knees and sit back into a squatting position toward the couch without actually sitting down. Try to stop before your butt touches the seat.

3. Stand up and repeat the exercise. Feel the contraction in your butt and thigh muscles.

Lean Machine Do two sets, 8 to 10 repetitions per set.

Muscle Maker Do two sets, 10 to 15 repetitions per set.

Fat Fighter Do two sets, 15 to 20 repetitions per set.

Couch Press

This is a great exercise for your chest and upper body.

1. Stand facing your couch. Put your arms in front of you on the seat cushions as you lower your body and place your feet straight back behind you, or in a modified kneeling position.

2. Bend your elbows and lower your chest toward the couch. Press back up to your starting position and repeat the exercise.

Lean Machine Do two sets, 8 to 10 repetitions per set.

Muscle Maker Do two sets, 10 to 15 repetitions per set.

Fat Fighter Do two sets, 15 to 20 repetitions per set.

Couch Dips

This exercise builds your upper-body strength.

1. Place your hands shoulder width apart on the edge of a couch. Your feet should also be shoulder width apart. Your butt is barely touching the edge of the couch and your body weight is supported by your arms.

2. Extend your elbows 90 degrees and raise your body as you extend your elbows. Don't lock your elbows. Feel the squeeze in the back of your arms. Imagine that you are wringing out a towel as you lift up your body.

3. Bend back down to starting position.

Lean Machine   Do two sets, 8 to 10 repetitions per set.

Muscle Maker   Do two sets, 10 to 15 repetitions per set.

Fat Fighter   Do two sets, 15 to 20 repetitions per set.

Couch Crunch

Feel your abs work!

1. Lie on the floor with your knees bent 90 degrees and place your feet on the couch. Put your hands behind your head with your fingers touching each other.

2. Slightly curl up toward the sofa. Feel the contraction in your abs as you squeeze those muscles. Slowly lower yourself toward the floor to starting position.

Lean Machine   Do two sets, 15 to 20 repetitions per set.

Muscle Maker   Do two sets, 15 to 20 repetitions per set.

Fat Fighter   Do two sets, 15 to 20 repetitions per set.

the houseclean pump

Housework can be part of your daily workout routine. Here are a few exercises that can help you fit in fitness even when it's your turn to clean.

Dishwashing Upper-Body Pump

1. Place your hands on the edge of the kitchen sink.

2. With a straight back, bend your elbows 90 degrees and position your feet a few inches away from the sink.

3. Bring your body in toward the sink as if you are doing a push-up. Then press yourself back up as you straighten out your arms. Keep your elbows slightly bent.

Lean Machine Do two sets, 8 to 10 repetitions per set.

Muscle Maker Do two sets, 10 to 15 repetitions per set.

Fat Fighter Do two sets, 15 to 20 repetitions per set.

Vacuum Lunge

1. Stand tall in neutral alignment with your feet shoulder width apart, holding on to the vacuum cleaner for support.

2. Step forward with one leg and place your full foot on the floor in front of you. As you step forward, your back leg will bend at the knee but your knee should not touch the floor. Push back and feel the squeeze in your legs and butt muscles. Stay in control. Imagine you are stepping over a small puddle of water. Be sure not to let your knees extend over your toes.

3. Switch legs and repeat.

Lean Machine Do two sets, 8 to 10 repetitions per set.

Muscle Maker Do two sets, 10 to 15 repetitions per set.

Fat Fighter Do two sets, 15 to 20 repetitions per set.

Avoid lunges if you have knee problems.

Upper-Body Laundry Challenge

Whether you do your laundry at home or at the Laundromat, you can take a few minutes to work your upper body.

Equipment needed: Laundry basket

Working muscles: Upper back, shoulders, arms, and chest

1. Stand tall in neutral alignment with your feet shoulder width apart. Your knees should be slightly bent.

2. Pick up your filled laundry basket or bag and hold it in front of you. Maintain this position for as long as you can. You will be using many of your upper-body stabilizing muscles. Beginners should strive to hold the position for 30 to 60 seconds. The more fit and the more advanced should be able to hold the position for 2 minutes or more. Each time you do your laundry, try to improve your time.

part three

the body noble lifestyle

12

noble nutrition

Clients are always asking me, "Derek, what diet do you like?" My response is that I don't like any of them!

I am against all weight-loss diets. When someone says they are going on a diet, what they are really saying is that they are going to eat differently than they normally eat for a while so that they can lose weight. The truth is, you'll lose weight on almost any diet, but few people actually stick to a diet once they've lost the weight. There's a better approach to maintaining a healthy weight so that you can have a strong, attractive body. It's commonsense eating.

I spend a good deal of my time teaching my clients to think about weight and fitness in a new way. My first task is to dispel unrealistic expectations. Although you can lose a lot of weight fairly quickly on a restrictive diet, much of what is lost is water weight, not the excess fat that you want to lose. You may weigh in lighter on the scale, but you still may look flabby and unfit. True fitness is a long-term goal—it won't happen overnight. To make permanent changes in your body, you must first make them in your mind. Get rid of your false beliefs about dieting. Get real. Think practical. Think common sense. If weight-loss diets really work, why do so many people bounce from diet to diet and why despite all this dieting are so many people still overweight?

The truth is, there is no secret to being fit and looking great. Your weight is directly related to how much you eat in relation to how much energy you burn. Think of your body as if it were a bank account. If you deposit more than you withdraw, you are going to gain weight. Find the right balance between food intake and activity level to achieve a healthy, attractive, strong body.

This doesn't mean that everyone can eat the same way and get the same results. Fat fighters may need to eat a bit differently than muscle makers or lean machines (and vice versa), but they still don't need to go on a diet. Beginning on page 174, you will find a basic eating plan for each of the three body types: lean machines, muscle makers, and fat fighters. Regardless of our body type, we all need to develop good eating habits that can last us for a lifetime so that we never have to go on a diet in the first place. My primary goal is to teach people how to *eat clean*. By eating clean, I mean choosing food as free of bad chemicals (such as pesticides or additives) as possible, prepared in a way that doesn't destroy vital nutrients or add a lot of fat and calories. Clean food is not smothered in sauce or floating in fat. It is high-quality, fresh food that is prepared quickly and simply but still tastes great. Once you understand the basic principles of eating clean, you will be able to make the right food choices for you, based on your likes and dislikes. The same principle applies whether you eat most of your meals at home, in restaurants, or at your desk at work.

I also teach people to *eat smart*. Smart eating means eating five times throughout the day—three meals and two snacks. It also means not eating a huge meal at night before you go to sleep, but distributing your calories more evenly throughout the day when you can burn them up. It's really that simple.

We all have foods that we love to eat, and some of them may not be that healthy. I find that if people try to completely eliminate their favorite forbidden food, they are more likely to fail. That's why I believe that once a week it's important to indulge in some of your favorite foods.

Have a sinfully rich dessert or eat an entrée that may be somewhat higher in fat than you would the rest of the time. Just don't make a habit of it. I call this the Noble Pleasure Response. Add this to your weekly program.

On the Body Noble Eating Plan, there are five food categories to choose from: protein, low-glycemic carbohydrates, high-glycemic carbohydrates (the glycemic index is a rating system for food based on how it affects insulin and blood sugar levels), healthy fats, and unhealthy fats. These foods are organized into meals that are both nutritious and satisfying. Beginning on page 176, you will find lists of recommended foods. To make it really easy, beginning on page 186, I provide a week's worth of menus so that you can see how it all fits together. I hope that once you understand the principles of eating clean, you'll be able to design your own program. That's why I call it flexible—I don't want everyone slavishly following the same program.

know your nutrients

There are two types of nutrients: macronutrients and micronutrients. Macronutrients include protein, fat, and carbohydrate. Macronutrients provide us with energy. Micronutrients include vitamins and minerals, which are also necessary for life but are consumed in small quantities. I recommend that people take a good vitamin and mineral supplement to make up for what may be missing from their food. At times, I recommend specific supplements to help improve your metabolism and promote fat burning. At the end of the day, it's the quality and quantity of the macronutrients you eat along with your fitness program that determine the shape of your body, not any magic pills you may be taking.

protein

Protein is found in both animals and plants and includes beef, pork, lamb, poultry, fish, game, soy, and dairy products. During digestion, food protein is broken down into amino acids. There are twenty different amino acids, of which eleven can be made by the body. The other nine, called essential acids, must be obtained through food. Animal protein contains all nine essential amino acids. Plant-based food, with the exception of soybeans and a few grains (such as quinoa), does not contain all nine essential amino acids. If you are a vegetarian who eats dairy products, you can easily compensate for what's missing in plant proteins by adding eggs and/or dairy foods (milk, low-fat cheese, yogurt, or protein powder) to your meal. If you are a total vegan—that is, you don't eat any animal food products—make a conscious effort to combine the right plant proteins in each meal to be sure that you are getting all your essential amino acids. For example, grains may have some of the essential amino acids, while legumes (lentils, black beans, pinto beans, almonds) and nuts may have others. Brown rice and beans, and a whole-grain almond butter sandwich are examples of combining foods to create meals of complete proteins. When two different foods combine to provide the nine essential amino acids, they are called complementing proteins.

Protein foods tend to fill us up quickly and keep us satisfied longer than carbohydrates. Many carbohydrates, when broken down in the body, are quickly converted into sugar, which triggers a sharp spike in the hormone insulin. This gives you that brief energy boost, or sugar high. The sugar is burned off quickly, however, and your insulin level drops, which leaves you feeling hungry. Proteins do not trigger as sharp a spike in insulin as do many carbohydrates and they take longer for the body to burn off, which keeps you feeling fuller for longer periods of time. That's why high-protein diets are so popular. Moreover, in the absence of carbohydrates, protein is readily burned off by the body and not stored as fat. A high-protein diet helps eliminate excess fat more quickly than a diet that includes a high amount of carbohydrates, but this doesn't mean that gorging on protein all day is particularly good for you. For one thing, many carbohydrates contain micronutrients that are missing from protein and are essential for good health. Second, protein tends to be higher in fat than carbohydrates, and not necessarily in healthy fat.

Protein foods (notably red meat and full-fat dairy products) are often a source of saturated fat, which is unhealthy in high amounts. High levels of saturated fat may promote heart disease and cancer. I don't recommend eating a diet high in saturated fat. You will notice that certain cuts of red meat are not on the protein list, such as brisket, prime rib, and short ribs. These cuts are high in saturated fat and should only be eaten rarely, if at all. Fortunately, there are lots of lean protein choices that are low in saturated fat, and those are the ones that I list as acceptable food choices. Poultry contains less saturated fat than red meat, and white meat turkey and chicken are great choices because they are very low in saturated fat. (Always remove the skin, since it is high in saturated fat.) Fish is also an excellent protein source because it is low in bad fat and contains omega 3 fatty acids, which are good for you.

As noted earlier, soy contains all nine essential amino acids and is a wonderful alternative to meat and other animal proteins. Soy protein has long been used as a meat substitute or meat extender, and it can be made into everything from veggie burgers to hot dogs to chili. The frozen food shelves of supermarkets and health food stores are packed with soy-based products. I invite you to try them. Soy food tends to be lighter and easier to digest. It is also a rich source of plant chemicals including protease inhibitors, which may inhibit the growth of cancerous cells. Soy also contains plant estrogen, which may relieve menopausal symptoms in some women. (However, plant estrogen may stimulate the growth of estrogen-sensitive breast tumors, so women who have a history of breast cancer or are at high risk of breast cancer should talk to their doctors before eating soy foods.) Tofu, or bean curd, is a mild-tasting, white, cheeselike cake made from soybeans. Tofu comes in many different forms and can be used in an infinite number of ways. It has little flavor of its own and soaks up any flavor that is added to it. It can be used as a cheese substitute in lasagna or a chicken substitute in stir fry dishes, or can be made into a mock egg salad with the right seasoning. While soy is a great alternative, it is best to eat a variety of different low-fat proteins.

carbohydrate

Carbohydrate is a general term for a wide range of foods including vegetables, fruits, grains, cereals, and legumes (beans). There are two types of carbohydrates: simple and complex. Simple carbohydrates include food made from refined white flour, such as commercially processed white bread, rolls, waffles, cakes, cookies, and junk food such as chips, candy bars, and so on. Complex carbohydrates include most fruits, vegetables, and legumes and food made from whole grains, such as whole-grain breads and pastas, and unprocessed cereals (such as steel-cut oatmeal). There is a significant difference in how simple and complex carbohydrates are digested by the body. Simple carbohydrates are broken down very rapidly in the bloodstream, causing a sharp spike in blood sugar and insulin, the hormone that controls sugar. They are rated high on the glycemic index, a system of rating food according to how it affects blood sugar and insulin levels. The problem with simple carbohydrates is that after the initial sugar-insulin spike, there is a sharp drop in your blood sugar, which will result in your feeling hungry very quickly. This often leads to craving more simple carbohydrates, which can lead to rapid weight gain. In contrast, complex carbohydrates are broken down more slowly by the body, creating a smaller rise in insulin and blood sugar. Complex carbohydrates also contain lots of healthy things such as fiber (which slows down the breakdown and absorption of carbs and can help stabilize blood sugar), vitamins, minerals, and other nutrients that are stripped from refined foods during processing.

Carbohydrates are essential for good health, but you need to eat the right ones in the right amounts. In my experience, people who follow very low carbohydrate diets run out of steam easily and just don't have enough energy to get through the day. Complex carbohydrates are an excellent source of energy, but you do want to burn them off. I recommend that people eat complex carbohydrates in the morning along with some protein to keep them going strong. I often start my day with a bowl of oatmeal (not instant) and an egg white omelet or a protein shake. (I allow myself six eggs a week, but limit egg yolks because they are high in saturated fat.) There is even a place for high-glycemic carbs in your diet—they really do provide an instant energy spurt—but only the right ones in small amounts. For example, a banana is a high-glycemic carb, but it is also an excellent source of potassium and other minerals, and can add wonderful flavor to a protein shake. A slice of cantaloupe, also a high-glycemic carb, is a refreshing dessert that is filled with phytonutrients, beneficial chemicals that are found only in fruits, vegetables, and fiber. In contrast, a doughnut is also a high-glycemic carb, but it doesn't have any of the vitamins or minerals found in bananas or cantaloupe. So choose your high-glycemic carbs wisely.

To make it easy for you, I have created my own version of the glycemic index and have divided carbohydrates into two categories: low-glycemic carbohydrates (the slow-burning kind) and high-glycemic carbohydrates (the fast-burning kind). In addition to considering the carbohydrate's effect on blood sugar and insulin levels, I also factor in the nutrient content of the food. For instance, on the standard glycemic index, yams would be considered a high-glycemic carbohydrate. On my list, however, I take into account that yams are packed with beta-carotene, a great source of vitamin A, and fiber and other nutrients, so I list yams as a low-glycemic carb. Most fruits and vegetables are listed under low-glycemic carbs; however, there are some notable omissions, including cooked carrots, bananas, white potatoes, and other starchy or very sweet fruits or vegetables that elicit a strong sugar-insulin response.

fat

When most of us hear the word "fat," we think in negative terms. We've all been told, fat makes you fat. Fat is bad for you. Don't eat fat. None of this is true. Fat is like any other nutrient. We need it to survive—even to thrive—but we also need to be careful about which types of fat we eat and how much of it we eat. If you don't believe that you must eat fat to be healthy, just look at people following very low-fat diets. Typically, their hair is dull and brittle, their nails are chipped, their skin is dry, and they don't have much energy. Fat provides the raw materials for cholesterol, which is made into hormones, and is the structure of cell membranes (the protective covering around cells). Your brain contains a high concentration of fat. And fat is required for the absorption of the fat-soluble vitamins A, D, E, and K.

There are four different types of fat found in food: monounsaturated fat, polyunsaturated fat, saturated fat, and trans fatty acid. Some types of fat are healthy and some are very unhealthy. Monounsaturated fat (omega 9 fatty acids), the kind found in olive, almond, hazelnut, macadamia, and grapeseed oils, is a healthy fat. It is rich in antioxidants, substances that protect us against free radicals, potentially dangerous chemicals produced by our bodies as a by-product of energy production. Excess free radicals are implicated in virtually every disease, from cancer to heart disease to arthritis.

Other healthy fats include two polyunsaturated fats that are so important that they are called essential fatty acids. These include omega 3 fatty acids and omega 6 fatty acids. Your body needs them to function but can't produce them and must obtain them through food. Omega 3 fatty acids are found primarily in fatty fish (such as salmon, mackerel, albacore tuna, and sardines) and in the egg yolks of specially raised chickens that are fed a diet rich in omega 3 fatty acids. Omega 3s are especially important for your brain, and low levels have been linked to depression and learning problems. Contrary to the myth that eating fat makes you fat, several studies have shown that omega 3 fatty acids promote fat burning and muscle production. The right fat can turn your body into a fat-burning machine! Omega 6 fatty acids are found in nuts, vegetable oils, and grains. Most people eat enough omega 6 fatty acids, although not necessarily the right kind. They may be missing one type of omega 6 called gammalinoleic acid, or GLA, which is a natural antiinflammatory. Good sources of GLA include walnuts, avocados, and seeds. Heat, light, and oxygen destroy essential fatty acids.

What are the bad fats? Saturated fat, which is found in red meat (beef and lamb), pork, and whole-fat dairy products, has been linked to an increased risk of heart disease, Alzheimer's disease, and possibly some forms of cancer. It should be eaten in limited amounts. Butter is a rich source of saturated fat, and should be used sparingly (a small pat is one serving). Trans fatty acids, a man-made fat, is the worst kind of fat and should be avoided. Many brands of margarine and cooking oils undergo a chemical modification called hydrogenation to extend their shelf life and make them easier to use in baking. This process creates trans fatty acids, a synthetic fat that increases the risk of heart disease, diabetes, and other health problems. Trans fats are a common ingredient in processed baked products, including bread, chips, frozen waffles and pancakes, cakes, and snack foods. Frying food at high temperatures (with the oil bubbling hot) will also create trans fats. To avoid trans fats, don't buy products that contain partially hydrogenated vegetable oil or partially hydrogenated vegetable shortening. Until recently, food manufacturers were not required to list trans fats on food labels. As of 2004, the FDA requires that trans fatty acids be listed on food labels. If you see that a product contains trans fats, don't use it. Some enlightened manufacturers have removed trans fats from their foods and proudly state the fact on their labels. And there are some new brands of margarine such as Smart Balance that don't contain any trans fats. Their main advantage is that they taste like butter without the saturated fat.

The Body Noble Eating Plan emphasizes healthy fats but also allows for some unhealthy fats (like saturated fat) because they are found throughout the food supply and are not harmful in small amounts.

eat more fiber

Fiber refers to food substances found in plants that are not digested or absorbed by the body. Fiber is found in fruit, vegetables, legumes, and unprocessed grains (not the refined white grain products sold in most supermarkets or in sugary, highly processed cereals). Ideally, people should eat around 30 grams of fiber a day, but most people following the typical North American diet eat less than half that amount. Fiber is essential for normal digestion, and one type of fiber—insoluble fiber, found in foods such as legumes, wheat bran, and fresh greens—speeds up the movement of food through your intestine. If you eat adequate amounts of insoluble fiber, you should never need a laxative. Another type of fiber, soluble fiber, found in foods such as apple, oat bran, and broccoli, can lower blood cholesterol levels and may protect against heart disease. Fiber also slows the breakdown of carbohydrates in the blood, preventing sudden spikes in blood sugar that can leave you ravenous within an hour or two after eating a high-sugar meal. Fiber also expands in your stomach, leaving you feeling full and more satisfied.

Eat lots of green vegetables and high-fiber fruits. Look for whole grains that have the highest fiber content. When you start reading labels, you'll see a big difference in the fiber content of similar foods. For example, some brands of refined, processed cereal contain less than 1 gram of fiber per serving, while some brands of whole grain, unprocessed cereal have as much as 9 grams of fiber per serving. For added fiber, sprinkle fiber flakes or bran on your morning oatmeal or drink one of the high-fiber Greens Powder drinks. They are also a great source of phyto-chemicals and fiber. Buy bread that contains 3 or more grams of fiber per slice; one sandwich adds up to 6 grams of fiber. Once you start becoming conscious of your fiber intake, you will easily find ways to boost the fiber content of your meals.

Tips on Buying Produce

- Buy sun-ripened, undamaged, fresh-looking produce. Hothouse produce just doesn't have the same taste. Bruising or excess handling can destroy vitamins, so don't buy beat-up-looking fruits or vegetables.

- Organic produce is the best, if you can find it. You'd be surprised how many supermarkets now have organic produce sections, but I don't expect you to travel miles out of your way to buy organic. The primary advantage of organic produce is that it is free of pesticides and other chemical additives that can form toxins in your body. The Department of Agriculture certifies organic products. Look for labels that say "100 percent organic." My favorite stores,

Whole Foods and Trader Joe's, offer excellent organic products and make shopping easy.

- Frozen produce is an excellent option for busy people. I always keep a bag or two of my favorite frozen mixed vegetables in the freezer, and cook them up at night with my protein for a quick meal. If you buy frozen vegetables or fruit, be sure that the produce is not clumped together in a solid block. That's a sign that the product has been defrosted and refrozen, which will destroy nutrients. Make sure you can feel the individual frozen pieces inside the package. You don't have to forgo organic if you use frozen products. Many health food stores and some supermarkets sell frozen organic products.

Tips on Preparing Produce

- All produce, organic or not, needs to be thoroughly washed. Even organic produce can contain harmful bacteria that can cause food poisoning. Many of the phytonutrients are concentrated in the skin of fresh fruits or vegetables, so try not to peel your produce. Instead, wash it well with a citrus produce wash (sold in supermarkets). Washing will remove most of the pesticides and other additives such as wax used to make skin shiny.

- Prepackaged cut-up fruits and vegetables or salad mix also need to be washed even if the package says that they have been prewashed. Salad mix in particular can harbor harmful bacteria, which can be eliminated by a careful washing. Packaged prewashed salad mix is usually dated because it can go bad. Don't use prewashed salad that has passed its expiration date—it can become a breeding ground for bacteria.

Tips on Cooking Produce

- Cook your vegetables as simply as possible. Steaming is the best way to preserve nutrients. Cut your vegetables into small, bite-size pieces. To steam vegetables, microwave or place them in a steamer basket (you can buy one at most supermarkets or houseware stores). Place an inch or so of water in a pot, place the basket inside the pot, cover, and let cook over a low flame. Most vegetables will take around three to five minutes, although others such as Brussels sprouts can take around fifteen minutes. Test with a fork for desired tenderness. Don't overcook your vegetables. It's best to eat them firm or al dente. They not only taste better, they also retain more nutrients.

- Stir-fry vegetables in a small amount of chicken broth or olive oil. You can also use a nonstick pan. Cook over a medium flame until the vegetables are tender, stirring often to make sure that they are cooked evenly.

- Cooking vegetables in the microwave is fine in a pinch, but keep in mind that microwaves can destroy B vitamins (such as folic acid). Be sure to use microwave cookware. Check your microwave instruction manual to see the correct cooking time for vegetables and the best cooking techniques for your model.

- For a treat, try grilling vegetables on an outdoor or indoor grill. Cut vegetables into bite-size pieces, brush a bit of olive oil on them, and cook them until they are tender. Mushrooms, peppers, and zucchini are great grilled.

Tips on Buying Meat, Poultry, and Fish

- Red meat (lamb and beef) and pork are high in saturated fat, so buy the leanest cuts possible. Cattle are often fed growth hormones and antibiotics to fatten them up and prevent disease. Unfortunately, these chemicals can be passed on to humans in the food supply, so whenever possible, try to buy hormone-free, antibiotic-free meat. Many supermarkets and health food stores carry these products.

- Game meats (buffalo, ostrich, and venison) are higher in omega 3 fatty acids and lower in saturated fat than beef or lamb. At one time it was hard to find game meats, but now they are carried by many supermarkets and health food stores. They taste a lot like beef, only they are lighter and leaner.

- Poultry (chicken and turkey) may also be fed growth hormones and antibiotics. Free-range, hormone- and antibiotic-free poultry is a good choice because it not only is chemical free but also contains higher levels of good fats.

- Buy the freshest fish possible. Avoid farm-raised fish since they are typically fed growth hormones or antibiotics. Use your nose to buy fish. Fresh fish doesn't smell fishy. Another way to tell if fish is fresh is to check that the eyes of the fish are clear, not scaly.

- Canned fish is fine. Keeping cans of salmon or tuna packed in water (not soybean oil) in your cupboard is an easy way to make sure you have access to fish if you can't get to the fish store or the supermarket.

Tips on Preparing Meat, Poultry, and Fish

- All meat, poultry, and fish should be baked, broiled, grilled, sauteed, or poached with little or no oil. For moisture and added flavor, baste red meat with broth and poultry and fish with lemon or orange juice.

- Trim meat of excess fat before cooking.

- Add 1 to 2 teaspoons of your favorite condiment (barbecue sauce, peanut sauce, mustard) after cooking to enhance flavor. Don't smother your food in fattening sauces. That's not clean eating!

- Indoor grills (like the George Foreman grill or the Hamilton Beach grill) are a great way to cook meat, poultry, and fish. They're not only more convenient and easier to use than outdoor grills, but are healthier. Grilling meat, a cooking method where food is exposed directly to the flame, produces cancer-causing chemicals in the smoke when the fat from the meat drips into the coals. Indoor grills allow for fat drainage into a special container without producing smoke. Furthermore, cooking meat at high temperatures—under an oven broiler or an outdoor grill—also produces cancer-causing substances within the meat itself. Indoor grills are specially designed not to exceed safe temperatures and should not produce these chemicals.

- A note for cooking novices: Food must be handled safely or you can get sick. Use a separate cutting board for meat and produce. Be careful about *not* reusing knives and utensils used to cut meat or poultry on vegetables or fruit before washing them first. Wash all cutting boards and utensils in hot, soapy water or in a dishwasher. Poultry can harbor salmonella, bacteria that can cause food poisoning. Be extra careful about handling poultry and washing down any utensil or surface that comes in contact with raw poultry.

- Use a meat thermometer to make sure that meat and poultry are cooked through. The Center for Science in the Public Interest recommends cooking beef to 160 degrees; poultry to 185 degrees; and lamb, veal, and pork to 170 degrees. You can get salmonella from eggs, too, so be sure to cook eggs thoroughly. Quickly refrigerate cooked meats after serving them.

Tips on Buying Dairy

- Full-fat dairy products are high in saturated fat, which is the toughest fat to burn. Fat fighters should stick to nonfat dairy products; muscle makers and lean machines can use low-fat (1 percent) dairy products.

- Butter is rich in saturated fat. If you love butter, have an occasional pat (less than a teaspoon) but do not gorge on it.

are you milk intolerant?

Dairy foods are not for everyone. About 50 million Americans suffer from lactose intolerance, the inability to digest high amounts of lactose, the predominant sugar found in milk. If you experience gas, bloating, diarrhea, or nausea after consuming a dairy product, chances are you're one of them. If you have this problem, it's best to avoid dairy foods or to stick to lactose-reduced products. Lactaid pills that contain lactose may help enhance the absorption of dairy products for some people. If you are lactose intolerant, you don't have to feel deprived. Soy milk, rice milk, and almond milk are excellent substitutes for dairy and can be used in milk and cereal. There are five brands of soy cheese, soy yogurt, and soy ice cream that can pass for the real thing.

are you gluten intolerant?

Gluten is a protein found in wheat, rye, barley, and oats. Many people have difficulty digesting gluten and experience gas and bloating when eating these foods. Wheat is a particular offender. When clients tell me that they are experiencing bloating or gas for no apparent reason, I often suggest that they try avoiding gluten foods for a while. There are some wonderful gluten-free breads and muffins, including my favorite wheat and gluten-free products manufactured by Foods for Life, sold in many health food stores and supermarkets. Very often, symptoms disappear after making the switch. I have also found that gluten intolerance and lactose intolerance go hand in hand, and when people avoid both foods, their digestive problems are vastly improved. There are varying degrees of gluten intolerance. While some people may get a mild upset stomach from gluten, in its severest form, gluten sensitivity can be life threatening. If you have severe digestive symptoms, such as chronic diarrhea, abdominal pain, or unexplained weight loss, you should see your doctor. It could be that you are sensitive to gluten or have another medical problem.

what to drink?

My favorite beverage is pure water, preferably filtered by reverse osmosis or bottled by a reputable company. There is a great deal of chlorine and other chemicals in tap water, so I recommend not drinking it if possible. I fear that all these chemicals could have a detrimental effect on health long term. I do want you to drink eight full glasses of water daily. The human body is 70 to 80 percent water, and we need to replenish the water we lose in our daily living. If you don't like water or get bored with it, add a splash of fresh lemon, orange, or your favorite juice. A splash means just that—an ounce or two for flavor. Juice is high in sugar and calories. For a refreshing treat, try soaking cucumber slices in ice water. It gives the water a delicate flavor that makes it go down a bit more easily.

So-called sports drinks are not a substitute for water. Many are loaded with sugar and artificial flavors. The better brands contain sodium and potassium, two minerals lost in sweat that are important to replenish after a vigorous workout. I usually mix my favorite sports drink with water to cut down on sugar and I sip it during and after my workout when I get tired of plain water.

A cup or two of coffee or tea (especially green tea), is fine as long as you don't overdo the caffeine. It can make you very jittery and interfere with sleep.

Herbal teas are great. You can drink them all day as long as they are not sweetened or contain caffeine. I recommend peppermint and chamomile.

Wine, beer, and other spirits are okay as long as you follow my one or none rule. Don't have more than one drink a day. Alcohol can put on weight very quickly, and people often forget that beverages count in their daily calorie total. Two 5-ounce glasses of wine add up to an extra 200 calories daily. In most cases, if you consume an extra 200 calories every day, you are going to put on weight. Avoid mixed drinks, which tend to be high in sugar and even more calorie dense. Drink your liquor straight up or with a bit of club soda or water. (One drink means just that—one small shot glass of hard liquor, about 5 ounces of wine, or one 12-ounce serving of beer.)

Avoid sugary soda. You can drink diet soda if you must, but I'm not crazy about artificial sweeteners. Try club soda with a twist of lemon, lime, or orange. It's better for you.

sweeteners

My favorite sweetener is organic honey. It tastes great and contains healthful antioxidants. Don't overdo the honey, though—it is still a source of sugar and calories. Stick to a teaspoon of honey in your coffee or tea. Avoid aspartame and other artificial sweeteners. You don't need to fill your body with chemicals.

eat a noble portion

When I first moved to the United States from Canada, I was shocked at the supersized food portions doled out at restaurants. The typical meal could easily feed two if not more people! I just read about a fast-food restaurant offering a new burger made up of two-thirds of a pound of beef, several slices of cheese, and bacon. This megaburger weighs in at nearly 1,500 calories and a shocking 107 grams of fat, most of it saturated fat. And believe it or not, it's selling like hotcakes. Given the statistics on obesity in the United States, I have no doubt that people are supersizing their portions at home. Supersized portions create supersized bodies. More than half of all adults in North America are overweight, and nearly 25 percent are considered to be obese, that is, they weigh 20 percent or more over their ideal weight. Obesity is not just a cosmetic problem; it can increase the risk of serious health problems such as diabetes, heart disease, and dementia. One of the first things I teach new clients is what a healthy meal should look like on their plate. I literally draw a food map so that people can see what normal portions look like. I encourage them to eat food from all the major food groups—including proteins, carbohydrates and fat—and I teach them how to make the best choices from each group in the right amount for them.

Below are the appropriate portion sizes for everyone, regardless of body type.

Protein—What's a Portion?

1 Full Protein Portion = a piece of beef, lamb, pork, poultry, or soy food the size of the palm of your hand—the inner portion not including the fingers or thumb

1 Full Protein Portion = 1 scoop of protein powder in a shake

1 Full Protein Portion = a fist-size serving of yogurt or cottage cheese (about 8 ounces)

1 Snack Protein Portion = half a full protein portion (one-half the size of your palm) or half a protein bar

Carbohydrate—What's a Portion?

1 Low-Glycemic Carb Portion = the size of your entire hand, palm plus fingers and thumb

1 High-Glycemic Carb Portion = the size of half a low-glycemic carb (half the size of your palm)

Fat—What's a Portion?

1 Fat Portion = 1 teaspoon of oil

1 Fat Portion = 1 pat of butter

eating guidelines for lean machines

If you are a lean machine, follow these eating guidelines:

You should eat 5 times daily—3 full meals and 2 snacks.

Eat 3 full servings of protein and 2 snack-size servings of protein daily.

Eat 4 servings of low-glycemic carbs and 3 servings of high-glycemic carbs daily.

Eat 4 servings of healthy fat and no more than 1 serving of unhealthy fat.

If you are hungry between meals, eat an extra snack protein serving.

eating guidelines for muscle makers

If you are a muscle maker, follow these eating guidelines.

> You should eat 5 times daily—3 full meals and 2 snacks.
>
> Eat 3 full servings of protein and 3 snack-size servings of protein daily.
>
> Eat 3 servings of low-glycemic carbs and 2 servings of high-glycemic carbs daily.
>
> Eat 3 servings of healthy fat and no more than 1 serving of unhealthy fat.
>
> If you are hungry between meals, eat an extra snack protein serving.

eating guidelines for fat fighters

If you are a fat fighter, follow these eating guidelines.

> You should eat 5 times daily—3 full meals and 2 snacks.
>
> Eat 2 full servings of protein and 2 snack-size servings of protein daily.
>
> Eat 3 servings of low-glycemic carbs and 2 servings of high glycemic carbs daily.
>
> Eat 2 servings of healthy fat and no more than 1 serving of unhealthy fat.
>
> If you are hungry between meals, eat an extra snack protein serving.

customizing the body noble eating plan

On the food lists that follow, you will see a wide selection of food choices to suit most palates. The food lists are divided into the following categories: protein, low-glycemic carbs, high-glycemic carbs, healthy fats, and unhealthy fats. Use these lists to help you put together your daily meals. I offer sample menus that are a reflection of how I eat for those of you who may want them.

Protein

BEEF

Beef tenderloin	Ground sirloin, lean or extra-lean (93% lean or more)	Round steak
Ground round, lean or extra-lean (93% lean or more)	Filet mignon	Roast beef
	Flank steak	Sirloin steak
		Veal roast
		Veal chop

LAMB

Chop	Roast	Leg

PORK

Canadian bacon (uncured, no nitrites or nitrates)	Lean ham (boiled or canned)	Loin chop
		Pork tenderloin

POULTRY

Chicken, white meat (skin removed)	Turkey, white meat (skin removed)	Ground turkey, low-fat
Cornish hen (skin removed)	Ground chicken	

GAME

Buffalo	Ostrich	Rabbit
Duck (drained of fat, skin removed)	Pheasant	Venison

SOY

Soy burgers	Soy dogs	Tofu

DAIRY

Eggs

Egg whites

Feta cheese

1% low-fat or nonfat cottage cheese

1% low-fat or nonfat yogurt

1% low-fat or nonfat cream cheese

1% low-fat or nonfat sour cream

1% low-fat ricotta

1% low-fat cheese

skim milk (one cup)

DAIRY SUBSTITUTES

Soy milk

Rice milk

Almond milk

FISH

Bass

Bluefish

Cod

Flounder

Haddock

Halibut

Lobster

Salmon (canned in water or fresh)

Sardines

Scallops

Shrimp

Swordfish

Tilapia

Trout

Tuna (canned in water or fresh)

Turbot

Whitefish

DELI MEATS

Sliced fresh chicken

Sliced fresh turkey

Sliced fresh roast beef

PROTEIN SUBSTITUTES

Protein powder

Low-carb protein bar

NUTS AND SEEDS

Almonds

Almond butter

Brazil nuts

Raw cashews

Macadamia nuts

Raw pumpkin seeds

Walnuts

Low-Glycemic Carbohydrates

VEGETABLES

Asparagus

Bamboo shoots

Bean sprouts

Bell peppers

Bok choy

Broccoli

Brussels sprouts

Cabbage

Carrot (a small amount of grated raw carrot sprinkled in salad)

Cauliflower

Celery

Eggplant

Endive

Garlic

Kale

Leeks

Mushrooms

Mustard Greens

Onions

Radishes

Salad mix

Scallions (green onions)

Snow peas

Spinach

String beans

Sugar snap peas

Summer squash

Sweet potatoes

Turnips

Watercress

Water chestnuts

Yams

Zucchini

LEGUMES

Chickpeas

Dried beans (any kind)

Hummus (mashed chick pea salad, homemade)

Kidney beans

Lentils

Refried beans

Split peas

Soybeans

FRUITS

Apple

Apple juice

Avocado

Blackberries

Blueberries

Cherries

Dried apricots

Grapes

Grapefruit

Kiwi

Lemon

Lime

Orange

Pear

Peach

Raspberries

Strawberries

Tomato

All-Bran

Basmati rice

Bran flakes

Bread crumbs made from whole wheat bread

Brown rice

Bran bread

Buckwheat

Kamut

Oatmeal, slow cooking (not instant)

Pumpernickel bread

Quinoa

Rye bread

Spelt

Tortilla wrapper whole wheat, high-fiber, or low-carb

Whole wheat pasta

Whole wheat bread

Whole wheat pizza crust (thin only!)

Wild rice

High-Glycemic Carbohydrates

VEGETABLES

Acorn squash

Beets

Cooked broad beans

Cooked carrots

Corn

Parsnips

Peas

Pumpkin

White potatoes

FRUIT

Banana

Cantaloupe

Honeydew melon

Plum

Pineapple

Watermelon

GRAINS

Bread (any bread or rolls made from white flour)

Bread crumbs made from white bread

Commercial cereals (any refined, presweetened cereal)

Chips

Cookies

Couscous

Crackers (any crackers made from white flour)

Rice cakes

Snack foods (baked or fried chips, pretzels, popcorn, etc.)

White pasta

White rice

MISCELLANEOUS

Sorbet | Table sugar | Processed maple syrup

Fats

GOOD FATS

Almond oil | Low-fat or nonfat mayonnaise | Soy mayonnaise (made from soy, not eggs)
Grapeseed oil | Macadamia oil | Walnut oil
Hazelnut oil | Olive oil |

UNHEALTHY FATS

Full-fat cheese

Full-fat ice cream

Margarine made from hydro-genated oils

Most processed vegetable oils (corn oil, peanut oil)

Full-fat mayonnaise

CONDIMENTS

(You can use 1 tablespoon of any condiment per meal—it doesn't count!)

A-1 sauce | Fat-free salad dressing | Organic honey
Barbecue sauce | | Relish
Canadian maple syrup | Honey mustard | Soy mayonnaise
Dijon mustard | Light peanut sauce dressing | Tabasco sauce
Fat-free mayo | | Specialty sauces
 | Marinade | Worcestershire sauce

eating out the noble way

Follow the basic eating plan whether you are eating at home or eating out. It doesn't matter whether you're in a fast-food restaurant or the priciest place in town, I guarantee that you will be able to stick with the program. It's all about making the right food choices wherever you are.

Restaurant portions are often enormous, much more than you should eat at one sitting. Don't be afraid to ask for a doggie bag to take the leftovers home for the next day. Eat leftovers for breakfast or take them to work for lunch. Make sure that you order your food cooked clean, without heavy sauces. Ask for fish, chicken, or lean cuts of beef, lamb, or pork grilled, baked, or poached in as little oil as possible. Don't order anything fried. You don't have to forgo flavor—order sauce on the side and use it sparingly.

My favorite salad dressing is balsamic vinegar with a touch of olive oil. Many restaurants will bring you a bottle of vinegar and olive oil so you can mix your own. That way you don't go overboard on fat.

Try to skip the bread basket—it's usually filled with flat-tasting white rolls. If you can't resist, one roll counts as one high-glycemic carb. But wouldn't you rather save your high-glycemic carb for something better, like mashed potatoes or pasta?

If you love dessert, split one dessert with someone else at the table. I do at least once a week so I don't feel deprived.

I cook a lot at home, but I also eat a few meals out every week. Here's what I order at my favorite restaurants.

Chinese Cuisine   Chinese food can be great for you or it can be terrible—it all depends on how it's prepared. When I eat at a Chinese restaurant, I never order anything deep-fried. Instead, I order a fresh vegetable spring roll (either in lettuce or a non-fried wrapper) with a bowl of fresh chicken soup and Asian vegetables. If I want heartier fare, I ask for lightly sauteed or steamed chicken or fish over Chinese greens and broccoli. I always ask for brown rice and I wash it all down with a cup of black or green tea.

Thai Cuisine   Thai food can make a wonderful clean meal or it can be dripping in heavy peanut sauce. I order skewers of grilled chicken or shrimp and ask for the sauce on the side. I dip just enough for flavor but not so much that it adds excess fat and calories. Thai restaurants usually offer lots of fresh salads and vegetables in tangy dressing. Once again, ask for the dressing on the side. Thai chicken soup with fresh vegetables makes a wonderful one-dish meal. I end my meal with a cup of fragrant jasmine tea.

The Deli   Just the word "deli" conjures up images of overstuffed pastrami sandwiches and french fries, but it doesn't have to be that way. Many delis offer a soup and sandwich special—half a sandwich with a bowl of soup. I order turkey breast or lean roast beef on multigrain or rye bread with Dijon mustard and a bowl of lentil or bean soup. I splurge on the half-sour pickles, and I don't even miss the pastrami. I drink iced tea or some seltzer with a spritz of lemon.

Mexican Cuisine   I love Mexican food and eat it often, but it can be high in bad fat if you're not careful. If you order guacamole (avocado dip), basically a healthy fat, don't wreck it by eating it with high-glycemic chips that are loaded with unhealthy trans fatty acids. Ask for fresh vegetables for dipping instead of chips. For a main course, I order the chicken or beef burrito without cheese or sour cream and an ice tea. If you can't stand the idea of eating your burrito naked, ask for a small portion of cheese or sour cream on the side, and use it sparingly.

Italian Cuisine   Italian food has become synonymous with pasta, but that's the one dish I never order at an Italian restaurant because it is usually made from white flour. When I crave pasta, I cook my own whole-grain high-protein pasta at home. Instead of pasta, I feast on fresh fish or chicken lightly sauteed in olive oil with some lemon, garlic, and herbs. Italian chefs make terrific vegetables such as broccoli, spinach, steamed escarole, or broccoli rabe sauteed lightly in olive oil with garlic. I treat myself to a glass of red wine (which is higher in antioxidants than white wine) and I feel full and happy.

Greek Cuisine   The Greeks have a great way of mixing clean protein with fresh vegetables and making it look fancy. One of my favorite dishes is shish kabob, skewers of beef, lamb, or chicken with vegetables such as onions, peppers, mushrooms, and tomatoes. I ask the waiter to hold the rice, and instead order a salad to go along with my meal. I do indulge in one high-glycemic carb—a slice of warm pita bread. For my beverage, I order sparkling water with a twist of lemon.

The Steak House   Stick to a leaner cut of beef such as filet mignon or sirloin, and enjoy it with fresh vegetables. Watch out for steak-house portions—they tend to be huge. So ask for a doggie bag and use the leftover steak in a salad the next day. If you can't imagine visiting a steak house without enjoying an onion ring or a double-stuffed baked potato, you can save up your daily allotment of high-glycemic carbs for this indulgence. Just watch your portion size.

Diner Breakfast   Order a vegetable omelet with rye toast (without butter) and a cup of black tea with lemon and honey, or iced tea.

fast-food restaurants

It's easy to follow the Body Noble Eating Plan even if your only option is a fast-food restaurant. Here's what I order for a quick bite on the road.

McDonald's or Burger King   Try the grilled chicken sandwich with barbecue sauce, lettuce, and extra tomatoes. If you crave beef, order two burgers (no mayo), and place both patties on half of a hamburger bun. Skip the fries and order a side salad with low-fat dressing. Drink water, unsweetened iced tea, or diet soda if you must—although I don't like artificial sweeteners.

Carl's Jr.   Your best bet is the grilled chicken sandwich with unsweetened iced tea. Order a side salad with low-fat dressing.

Domino's   Order the thin-crust pizza with vegetable topping (such as mushroom, onions, peppers).

Subway   Order the six-inch chicken breast sub and load it up with vegetables. Use one of their low-fat dressings.

Taco Bell   The grilled chicken burrito is a good choice and it tastes great.

shake it up!

If you're in a hurry, a protein shake makes a wholesome meal or snack. There are lots of prepackaged, ready-made protein shakes on the market, but I don't like any of them. Most of them contain sweeteners and other chemicals, and I don't like the way they taste. You are better off buying pure whey protein powder and making your own shake in a blender. Whey is derived from milk protein and does not contain lactose, the milk sugar that is hard to digest. There are lots of whey protein powders on the market. My favorite Body Noble protein supplement is Protein Plus. Read product labels carefully! Some whey protein powders are pure protein, while others are loaded with sugar and artificial sweeteners, which you don't need. I especially don't like aspartame, an artificial sweetener that has found its way into many so-called health foods. Aspartame is an excitotoxin, a chemical that can cause neurological problems in susceptible people (everything from dizziness, headaches, and stomach aches to feeling jittery). If you want a sweet flavor, you can add a quarter cup of fresh berries or half a banana to your shake and have all the added benefits of real fruit. It's easy to make a protein shake. Use 1 scoop of protein powder for every 8 ounces of water or low-fat dairy soy, rice, or almond milk. Add fruit of your choice and 1 tablespoon of EFA oil and blend for 30 seconds. In less than a minute, you have a great meal or snack. A good whey protein powder should blend well and taste great.

food bars

There are more and more brands of food bars (also called protein bars or meal-replacement bars) popping up on store shelves daily. If you read the ingredients, you will see that most of them are little better than candy bars. Although they may boast a higher protein content than a candy bar, many brands contain a chemical feast of additives, sugar, saturated fats, sugar substitutes, and fillers. There are better ways to get protein! Furthermore, most of these bars taste awful. I can recommend only one brand that I particularly like—it's the Organic Food Bar. They offer several excellent bars; my favorite is made with organic almond butter. It has a wonderful smooth flavor, doesn't contain a lot of nasty additives, and contains healthy fat. You can buy Organic Food Bars at Trader Joe's or Whole Foods, or check out their Web site, www.organic foodbar.com. These bars make a great snack or a meal in a pinch.

spice it up

Eating clean doesn't mean you have to eat bland. I don't want you to smother your food in heavy sauces, but that doesn't mean I suggest that you eat flavorless food. I keep lots of dried herbs and spices on hand in my kitchen to enhance the flavor of food. Dried herbs and spices are also a great source of antioxidants.

Here's a list of herbs and spices that I keep in my cupboard at all times:

Basil

Black pepper

Cayenne pepper

Chili powder

Cinnamon

Cumin

Garlic powder (For a more intense flavor, I often use fresh garlic with garlic powder. Ditto for onions!)

Ginger powder

Curry powder

Dill, dried

Kosher salt (which has a coarser texture than regular salt)

Onion powder

Oregano

Rosemary

Sage

Thyme

Turmeric

body noble sample 7-day meal plans

Day 1

BREAKFAST

> 2 scrambled omega 3 enriched eggs
>
> 2 slices of turkey bacon
>
> 1 slice of whole-grain toast
>
> Herbal tea (unsweetened only!) or coffee with low-fat milk
>
> 1 cup of water

MORNING SNACK

> ½ protein bar
>
> 1 cup of water or herbal tea

LUNCH

> Grilled turkey burger on an open-face sandwich of whole-grain bread
>
> Mixed green salad with ½ sliced avocado, vine-ripened sliced tomato, 1 sliced raw carrot, dressed with 2 tablespoons of balsamic vinegar, 1 tablespoon olive oil
>
> 1 cup of water with a splash of cranberry juice

AFTERNOON SNACK

> 1 cup of skim, soy, almond, or rice milk
>
> 1 sliced pear

DINNER

> 1 serving of ground, low-fat beef sauteed with garlic and onions
>
> 1 cup of brown rice
>
> 1 cup of fresh steamed broccoli
>
> 1 glass of water with lemon or lime slices

DESSERT

> ½ cup of mandarin segments

Day 2

BREAKFAST

Smoothie to go (1 scoop of whey protein powder, ½ banana, ¼ cup blueberries, ¼ cup soy, skim, almond, or rice milk, 1 cup water, and 1 tablespoon essential fatty acid oil, mixed in blender for 30 seconds)

Herbal tea or 1 cup of coffee with low-fat milk

MORNING SNACK

½ handful of healthy nut mixture, including macadamia nuts, almonds, pumpkin seeds, raw cashews

1 cup of herbal tea

LUNCH

Grilled chicken breast salad (1 chicken breast, sliced over mixed greens, ½ sliced avocado, 1 vine-ripened tomato, 1 sliced carrot, with fat-free dressing of your choice)

1 slice of whole-grain bread

1 glass of iced tea

AFTERNOON SNACK

1 cup of soy, skim, almond, or rice milk

1 tablespoon of almond butter on 1 high-fiber Rye Krisp

DINNER

1 piece of fresh, grilled, or baked fish of your choice

½ cup of quinoa or brown rice

½ cup of steamed Brussels sprouts or other green vegetable

1 cup of water with a splash of juice

DESSERT

½ cup of fruit sorbet

Day 3

BREAKFAST

> ½ cup of high-protein, high-fiber multigrain cereal of your choice with ½ cup soy, skim, or almond milk and 1 scoop of whey protein powder
>
> ½ banana
>
> 1 cup of water or herbal tea
>
> 1 cup of coffee (if you must) with low-fat milk

MORNING SNACK

> 1 piece of fruit
>
> 1 tablespoon of almond butter
>
> Water with a splash of juice

LUNCH

> Grilled salmon (or canned salmon) over mixed greens with cranberries, currants, and sliced almonds; dress salad with 2 tablespoons of balsamic vinegar, 1 tablespoon olive oil
>
> Herbal tea

AFTERNOON SNACK

> Soy milk latte (1 cup of vanilla-flavored soy milk with a splash of decaffeinated coffee and a sprinkle of cinnamon)

DINNER

> Grilled turkey cutlet
>
> 1 cup of low-fat tomato soup
>
> ½ of a baked sweet potato
>
> 1 cup of frozen mixed vegetables
>
> 1 cup of water with lemon slices

DESSERT

> ½ cup soy ice cream
>
> Herbal tea

Day 4

BREAKFAST

> 2 high-fiber, omega 3–enriched buckwheat frozen waffles
>
> 2 tablespoons of maple syrup
>
> Herbal tea or coffee with low-fat milk

MORNING SNACK

> 1 bottle of commercial low-fat yogurt smoothie drink

LUNCH

> 1 tuna sandwich on a whole wheat bagel with lettuce, tomatoes, and low-fat mayonnaise
>
> 1 glass freshly squeezed orange juice

AFTERNOON SNACK

> ½ protein bar
>
> Herbal tea

DINNER

> 1 grilled pork chop
>
> 1 cup of cooked mixed Chinese greens and broccoli rabe sauteed with olive oil and 2 sliced garlic cloves
>
> 1 glass of red wine

DESSERT

> 1 low-fat biscotti
>
> Herbal tea

Day 5

Vegetable omelet (2 whole eggs, 1 tablespoon of feta or goat cheese, plus ½ cup of your favorite vegetables)

1 slice of high-fiber whole-grain bread

½ cup of grapefruit juice

Herbal tea or coffee with low-fat milk

MORNING SNACK

½ cup of low-fat yogurt

½ cup of sliced banana

LUNCH

1 bowl of turkey chili

1 slice of whole-grain, high-fiber bread

1 cup of water with a splash of juice

AFTERNOON SNACK

1 protein shake (mix 1 cup of skim, soy, or rice milk in a blender with 1 tablespoon of essential fatty acid oil and ½ cup of frozen fruit, blended for 30 seconds)

DINNER

Whole wheat penne with low-fat beef marinara sauce

Mixed green salad; dress salad with 2 tablespoons balsamic vinegar and 1 tablespoon of olive oil

1 glass of red wine

DESSERT

½ cup of fresh fruit sorbet

Day 6

BREAKFAST

2 hard-boiled eggs

1 slice whole-grain, high-fiber toast

½ cup freshly squeezed orange juice

Herbal tea or coffee with low-fat milk

MORNING SNACK

½ protein bar

Herbal tea

LUNCH

1 bowl of low-fat chicken soup with mixed vegetables

1 glass of iced tea with lemon

AFTERNOON SNACK

½ cup of low-fat cottage cheese

½ cup of blueberries

Herbal tea

DINNER

Low-fat turkey meatloaf

1 cup of frozen vegetables

½ cup of brown rice or quinoa

DESSERT

½ cup of low-fat vanilla yogurt and 2 tablespoons of low-fat granola

Day 7

BREAKFAST

$\frac{1}{3}$ cup cooked oatmeal mixed with $\frac{1}{3}$ cup soy, almond, or rice milk with a dash of cinnamon

Scrambled eggs made from $\frac{1}{4}$ cup of egg whites and 1 omega 3 enriched egg

$\frac{1}{2}$ cup of freshly squeezed orange juice

Herbal tea or coffee with low-fat milk

LUNCH

1 veggie burger

1 slice whole-grain bread

Sliced tomato and onion

Mustard and ketchup

Herbal tea

AFTERNOON SNACK

$\frac{1}{2}$ handful of healthy nuts

1 cup of water with a splash of juice

DINNER

Protein of your choice served with microwaved fresh or frozen vegetables

DESSERT

$\frac{1}{2}$ cup of soy ice cream

13

noble supplements

Would you like a pill that makes your body sexy and svelte practically overnight, relieves stress, gives you lots of energy, and even makes you smarter?

The answer, of course, is yes. Who wouldn't want a great body and a sharp mind without ever having to watch what you eat or whether you workout? Does such a pill exist? The answer, of course, is no.

Regardless of advertisements and commercials for supplements by manufacturers who claim that their products can melt away fat while you sleep and help you lose tons of weight without dieting, take it from an expert—me—they don't work; there are no shortcuts to fitness. If you want to look good, you have to do good things for yourself. You have to eat well, work out, and learn to cope with stress in a realistic way. There is a role for supplements in the Body Noble Program, but it is secondary to nutrition and exercise.

Based on questions from my clients, I know that there is a great deal of confusion about supplements. Before I tell you which supplements I recommend, I'm going to provide some basic information. The term "supplement" refers to a wide variety of products taken to enhance health, ranging from the standard vitamins and minerals to the more exotic phytochemicals and nutraceuticals.

There are thousands of nutritional supplements on the market, and in my opinion, most are unnecessary. Supplements cannot take the place of a healthy diet, and if you follow the Body Noble Eating Plan, you are giving your body what it needs in the form that nature intended—food! Don't think that by popping a vitamin pill you can eat junk food all day and not pay the consequences. I understand, however, that busy people often don't eat as well as they should, and also that we can't always count on the food that we eat to contain ample amounts of vitamins and minerals. Modern food processing techniques can strip food of vital nutrients, and so can shipping and sitting on grocery store shelves. Even cooking can destroy some vitamins. That is why I recommend that everyone take a multivitamin every day. I view it as an insurance policy to make sure that you are getting the vitamins and minerals that your body needs to function. (When it comes to supplements, I always err on the side of caution. Please check with your doctor before taking any supplements.) In addition, I recommend a few other key supplements that I feel can enhance a healthy lifestyle.

I have designed my own brand of supplements for Genuine Health for the three different body types: lean machine, muscle maker, and fat fighter. It's a high-quality, all-natural product line, and in the resource section I tell you where to buy it, as well as recommend other high-quality brands. This chapter provides a blueprint of a good supplement program, and you can purchase your products wherever it is most convenient for you.

take a good multivitamin

Most of the popular brands of multivitamins (such as Centrum, One-a-Day, Genuine Health Twinlabs, Solgar, Theragran, Olay, and house brands Vitamin Shoppe and General Nutrition Center) contain at the very least the DRI for each vitamin and mineral, that is, the Dietary

Reference Intakes as determined by the National Academy of Sciences (formerly known as the RDA). The DRIs are the absolute rock bottom amounts of each vitamin and mineral that are required to prevent nutritional deficiency disease, such as scurvy, which is due to a long-term severe lack of vitamin C, or rickets, which is due to a severe lack of B vitamins. Although the DRIs are very low, amazingly, many people do not even ingest tiny amounts of all these vitamins and minerals every day. For example, although most people in the developed world will get enough vitamin C to prevent scurvy—that is, they don't go for months without obtaining any vitamin C in their food—they may not get the full DRI for C or other vitamins and minerals on a daily basis. This may not result in scurvy, but chronically low vitamin C intake may harm their health in other ways. To me, taking a multivitamin to make sure that you are covering all your bases is just good common sense.

Should you take a high-potency multivitamin, that is, one that contains more than the DRIs? There is a growing consensus among scientists that the DRIs are outdated—that based on scientific studies, the optimal intake of certain vitamins should be higher. For example, depending on your age, or whether you smoke, the DRI for vitamin C is between 40 to 90 mg daily. It's true that ingesting the DRI for vitamin C will prevent scurvy, but it is probably not enough to ensure optimal health. Vitamin C is a very important antioxidant that protects against toxic chemicals called free radicals that are produced in the body as a natural by-product of energy production. Vitamin C is also essential for a strong immune system. Most nutritionists agree that the DRI for C is too low to achieve optimal health, and recommend much higher doses, ranging anywhere from 500 to 2,000 mg daily. If you work out a lot, or are under a great deal of stress, you should consider taking a high-potency multivitamin. The same is true for many other vitamins and minerals. Some good brands of high-potency multivitamins include Genuine Health, NOW, Nature's Way, and others.

Many brands also offer multivitamins that are targeted to specific markets. For example, some brands of multivitamins are marketed to men, and these often include a phytochemical called lycopene (naturally found in tomatoes) that may be good for prostate health. In contrast, vitamins marketed to women may include phytochemicals that are similar in action to estrogen (such as those found in soy foods), which may relieve menopausal symptoms. Depending on your age and stage of life, you may want to consider one of these specialty products.

Clients often ask me if it's possible to overdose on vitamins. The reputable brands of multivitamins, including the high-potency vitamins that are sold at major outlets, typically do not contain doses of any single substance that are high enough to cause harm. I strongly recommend against self-dosage, that is, taking supplements by the handful on the assumption that if a little is good, more is better. Some vitamins such as vitamins A, E, D, and K are fat-soluble, which means that they are stored in fat deposits throughout the body. If taken in excess, these vitamins can be toxic. Even some water-soluble vitamins can be dangerous in very high doses. In theory, water-soluble vitamins that are not used by the body are eliminated in urine, but at times, too much may be absorbed by the body. For example, taking excess amounts of B vitamins can cause nerve damage. Your best bet is to stick with premixed formulas of multivitamins sold in major health food stores, pharmacies, or major discount stores.

There are numerous brands of multivitamins on the market. I urge you to find a brand of multivitamin that does not contain any artificial coloring, preservatives, or other unnecessary chemicals. Some multivitamins may contain ingredients you don't need. For example, men who are at risk of heart disease should probably not take extra iron unless told to do so by their physicians, because it may increase their risk of developing the disease. Women who are postmenopausal should also avoid taking extra iron for the same reason, but premenopausal women and teenage girls often need extra iron, especially if they work out a lot, because strenuous exercise can deplete iron stores. Furthermore, some supplements may not interact well with some prescription medication you may be taking. Once again, I urge you to check with your physician before taking a multivitamin or any other supplement.

> **Noble Tip**
>
> Take your supplements with food for better absorption and to avoid stomach upset.

Your multivitamin can't work if you don't take it. I take my vitamins in the morning with breakfast. I leave them out in an obvious place so I don't forget to take them.

In some cases, I recommend a few additional supplements along with a multivitamin.

calcium: an essential mineral

Calcium is essential for strong bones, and most women don't get enough of this vital nutrient. Women should get about 1,000 to 1,500 mg of calcium daily, but most don't. Anyone over fifty, male or female, should be sure to get 1,000 mg of calcium daily to avoid thin, brittle bones that can lead to osteoporosis. Calcium has other benefits: It may protect against colon cancer by reducing the risk of colon polyps, benign growths that can turn cancerous. Good food sources of calcium include low-fat dairy products, broccoli, kale, and canned salmon with bones. It would be great if you could get it in your food, but you shouldn't count on it. If your multivitamin doesn't contain enough calcium (and many don't), be sure to take a calcium supplement.

antioxidants

When you exercise—especially when you're doing cardio—your heart and lungs work harder to get oxygen and blood circulating throughout the body. As a result, your heart muscle gets more fit and so does the rest of your body. All of this is good for you, yet there is a negative side to exercise. While you're doing all that huffing and puffing, you are burning more oxygen to make energy, which means your body is producing more free radicals. What's so bad about free radicals? Free radicals are unstable oxygen molecules that in limited amounts are actually useful. For example, immune cells produce free radicals to kill bad stuff like bacteria and viruses that you don't want in your body. In excess, however, free radicals can be harmful. Because they are unstable, free radicals are constantly bonding with other molecules, which is bad because chemical reactions produce heat. As a result, too much free radical activity can harm healthy cells and organs, including your heart, your brain, and even your joints. Free radical damage has been implicated in virtually every disease from heart disease to cataracts to Alzheimer's disease to arthritis. Production of free radicals can be accelerated by chemicals found in the environment, toxins in food, smoke, smog, pollutants in the environment, and even UV rays emitted by the sun. The body has its own method of dealing with free radicals. It produces antioxidants such as glutathione and coenzyme Q10 to defuse free radicals and keep them under control. Vitamins C and E, which can only be obtained through food and supplements, are also powerful antioxidants. So are many of the wonderful phytochemicals found in fruits and vegetables. Most multivitamins fall short of antioxidants, which is why I recommend that everyone take an additional antioxidant supplement daily. Look for an antioxidant supplement that includes at least 1,200 mg of vitamin C and 400 IU of vitamin E daily.

essential fats

I recommend taking 1 tablespoon daily of a high-quality oil that contains essential fatty acids often missing from food. You need essential fats to repair nails, skin, and hair follicles and to burn fat. There are several good oils on the market, including omega 3s, UDO oil, flaxseed oil, and grapeseed oil. You can find a good oil at most health food stores and even some supermarkets. Flaxseed oil is the most fragile of the three oils, and should be refrigerated. It can go rancid very easily. All oil should be stored in a cool, dark place away from direct light. I usually put a tablespoon of either of these oils (I keep all three at home) in my protein shake daily. You can sprinkle the oil on your cereal or over vegetables, or use it in your salad dressing. I often mix grapeseed oil with balsamic vinegar in my salads.

As mentioned in chapter 12, Noble Nutrition, omega 3 fatty acids are also important for optimal health and are found in foods such as fatty fish and omega 3 enriched eggs, but I recommend that you also take a supplement. Many supplements derived from fish oil may contain mercury and other pollutants, so be sure to buy a product that specifically says it has been purified of any heavy metals. My favorite brands are Genuine Health, Spectrum, Whole Foods Private Label, Country Life, and Solaray. Look for an omega 3 fatty acid supplement containing around 360 mg of EPA and 120 mg of DHA per capsule. Take 2 capsules daily.

the fat burners

Fat burners are supplements that promote fat burning in the body, and while I don't necessarily recommend them for everybody, I do believe that they can be particularly useful for fat fighters. Some of these fat burners may already be in your multivitamin, so please read the label, and if your multi is missing these supplements or does not contain enough of them, consider buying additional supplements. I recommend a lipotrophic formula that contains most of these supplements.

Vitamin B_6   Also called pyridoxine, B_6 is important for the processing and metabolism of proteins, fats, and carbohydrates. Vitamin B_6 comes in doses ranging from 50 mg to 200 mg. I include 40 mg of B_6 in my multivitamin, and add an additional 10 mg to my lipotrophic formula, resulting in an intake of 50 mg of B_6 daily. Very high doses of B_6 (2,000 mg) can be toxic, so follow my advice and don't overdo it. I recommend taking 50 mg of vitamin B_6 daily.

L Carnitine   Carnitine is an amino acid–type substance found in the body and in food, primarily red meat. Carnitine is essential for the production of energy by the energy-producing part of your cells called mitochondria. Carnitine is often compared to the fuel pump in an automobile. Your body can have all the essential ingredients to make energy, but without carnitine, they cannot get into the mitochondrial engines where energy conversion takes place. Carnitine is also necessary for fat metabolism. Intense exercise produces a dramatic decline in carnitine in the body. Many athletes take carnitine to improve their performance and help create that "supercut" sculpted look. I recommend using carnitine sold in the form of L-carnitine or acetyl-L-carnitine in health food stores and pharmacies. I recommend taking either form of carnitine before and immediately following your cardio workouts. Take 300 mg of L-carnitine daily.

Inositol   Inositol is a form of the B vitamin niacin. Inositol is often recommended to people with heart disease because it helps to lower cholesterol and reduce the levels of other fats in the body. I recommend it for people who need to lean down. Don't use regular niacin! It can cause itching, flushing, and even liver damage. Inositol, especially in the dose that I recommend, is a safer form of niacin and usually doesn't cause any of these side effects, but once again, check with your physician before using this supplement. I recommend taking 250 mg of inositol daily.

Choline   Choline is another B vitamin that works with inositol to help the body burn up fat so it doesn't end up in places where you don't want it. Choline also helps to relieve stress, which is especially important for people who may eat excessively when they are under duress. At the same time, choline may also help improve mental performance. It is used by the brain to make acetylcholine, which is involved in memory and other important brain functions. I recommend taking 250 mg of choline daily.

L-glycine   L-glycine is an amino acid, a building block of protein, that promotes healing of muscle by delivering more creatine to muscle fibers. As many of you know, creatine is an important protein for muscle development and energy production. (Creatine is also sold separately as a supplement primarily for athletes who need to bulk up.) Glycine stimulates the release of glycogen, which is stored in muscles as an energy reserve. I recommend taking 500 mg of L-glycine daily.

L-methionine   L-methionine is an amino acid that helps break down fat. Methionine is essential for the production of creatine, which is necessary for muscle growth and energy production. Methionine also appears to boost levels of glutathione, an important antioxidant in the body that is depleted during times of intense physical activity. I recommend taking 250 mg of methionine daily.

Trimethyglycine   TMG is an amino acid that is essential for a process in the body known as methylation, an on/off switch that triggers hundreds of reactions in the body that are key to our health and well-being. Suffice it to say that methylation is as vital to our survival as breathing. The methylation of protein is key to the growth and repair of all cells in the body, and that includes muscle cells, your body's primary fat burners. I recommend taking 500 mg of TMG daily.

cure for achy joints

Arthritis is caused by the wearing down of cartilage, the protective covering that cushions bones and allows joints to move smoothly. As the cartilage wears down, bone rubs against bone, and that can be very painful. Symptoms of arthritis include stiffness, swelling, and joint pain, especially in the hips and knees. Arthritis is not just an old person's problem; by age fifty, at least half of all adults are affected by degenerative joint changes. You know that knee that aches all the time? That's the beginning of arthritis. At any age, athletes, especially runners and weight lifters, are at risk of developing arthritis because of chronic stress on their joints. That's one of the reasons I'm so opposed to people beating up their bodies and it's why I favor working with enough resistance to get results but not so much resistance that you are damaging your joints. My motto is: If it hurts, don't do it. The standard treatment for arthritis is to take a drug to control pain, usually a nonsteroidal antiinflammatory medication such as ibuprofen or naprosyn, but not to do anything about the underlying problem—cartilage degeneration. Two supplements— glucosamine and chondroitin—appear to address both problems. These supplements not only relieve the pain of arthritis for many people, but may help regenerate cartilage. I recommend that everyone over forty take glucosamine and chondroitin to protect against arthritis.

Chondroitin attracts fluid to cartilage, providing shock absorption for the surrounding bones and bathing the joint in healing nutrients. Glucosamine may actually stimulate the growth of new cartilage. These supplements work in synergy with each other and should be taken together for best results. I recommend two 500 mg capsules of each of glucosamine and chondroitin daily, or you can buy a combination product with the right amount of glucosamine and chondroitin.

14

strengthening
your weak links

When I evaluate new clients, I routinely ask them about any joint problems that may interfere with their workouts. In their eagerness to begin the Body Noble Workout, they typically tell me that they're fine. When I question them further, however, I often discover a potential weakness that could result in injury if they do not exercise with proper caution. If you have any orthopedic concerns such as arthritis, or a preexisting injury such as a sprained ankle, a tennis elbow, or a dislocated knee joint, it doesn't mean that you can't work out, but it does mean that you may have to modify one or more of the exercises so that you don't overtax the weak link or aggravate an existing injury. Over time, if you are diligent about following the Body Noble Method, your weak links will strengthen and very often become less of a problem. If you ignore your weak links, however, just the opposite may happen. You may sustain an injury that prevents you from working out for weeks or even months. The first step is to identify any weak links that could be interfering with your ability to achieve your Body Noble.

Do you know your weak links? Please take the following short quiz to determine if you have a problem that may need special attention.

When you have completed the questionnaire, turn to page 206 to help interpret your results. Once you have identified your weak links, please turn to page 208 for advice on how to work out safely and effectively.

where are your weak links?

1. Have you ever sustained an injury on any of the following parts of your body? Think all the way back to high school . . .

    a) Lower back ____

    b) One or both knee joints ____

    c) Neck or shoulders ____

    d) One or both hip joints ____

    e) One or both ankles ____

    f) One or both wrists ____

2. Which places in your body cause you the most discomfort?

    a) Lower back ____

    b) One or both knee joints ____

    c) Neck or shoulders ____

    d) One or both hip joints ____

    e) One or both ankles ____

    f) One or both wrists ____

3. Do you have restricted motion in any of these areas of your body?

    a) Lower back ____

    b) One or both knee joints ____

    c) Neck or shoulders ____

    d) One or both hip joints ____

    e) One or both ankles ____

    f) One or both wrists ____

4. When you wake up in the morning, do any of your joints ache?

   Yes _____ No _____

5. Do any of your muscles ever feel stiff?

   Yes _____ No _____

6. Do you get lower back pain?

   Yes _____ No _____

7. Can you touch your toes when you bend over while standing or sitting?

   Yes _____ No _____

8. Do you spend a lot of time sitting in your car?

   Yes _____ No _____

9. Do you have swelling anywhere in your body?

   Yes _____ No _____

10. Do your knees hurt when you walk down stairs?

    Yes _____ No _____

11. Do you suffer from headaches?

    Yes _____ No _____

12. Do you spend a lot of time at your computer?

    Yes _____ No _____

13. Do your shoulders and back hurt if you lift things overhead?

    Yes _____ No _____

14. Are you flexible?

    Yes _____ No _____

15. Do you regularly take antiinflammatory medication, such as aspirin, ibuprofen, or naprosyn?

    Yes _____ No _____

16. Do you routinely see a chiropractor?

    Yes _____ No _____

understanding your answers

Question 1   Forgot about that old injury, didn't you? The purpose of question 1 is to remind you of any injury that you may have sustained through the years. If you have injured any of the listed areas, please follow my workout advice for the related joint that I share later in this chapter.

Question 2   This question will help you identify any weak joints in your body that may be causing you pain or discomfort. If you have discomfort in any one or more of the body parts listed, please follow my workout advice later in this chapter.

Question 3   If your movement is restricted—if you have limited range of motion in a particular area of your body—it's a sign that you have a joint problem. People with tightness in their joints, or limited mobility, are more prone to injury doing everyday activities and when they are working out.

Question 4   Joint pain or ache upon rising in the morning is a sign of arthritis, the wearing down of the protective layer of cartilage that lines the joints that keeps your bones from rubbing against each other. There is absolutely no reason that people with arthritis should not work out, but check with your physician first.

Question 5   Stiff muscles are a sign of tightness in your muscles and joints. You need to be vigilant about stretching and maintaining flexibility.

Question 6   If you have lower back pain, you need to strengthen your abdominal muscles, those core muscles that support your back and upper torso. In addition, tight hamstring muscles can also cause lower back pain, so be sure to keep your hamstring muscles strong and flexible.

Question 7   If you can't touch your toes, it's a sign that your hamstrings are tight, which will make you more likely to develop a back or knee injury. Please do your stretching exercises every day to make those hamstrings more flexible.

Question 8   If you spend a lot of time sitting in your car, chances are you may have lower back problems. Think about it: Does your back ache, especially after you've been sitting in the car for a long time? Do you often feel stiff, especially in the legs and lower back? If you do, please follow my advice for people with back problems later in this chapter.

Question 9   I can't tell you how many times people tell me that they don't have any problems, but their knees swell up every night. Swelling is a sign of inflammation, and inflammation is a sign of injury. Applying ice for 10 minutes at a time to the swollen area can help relieve inflammation. Be careful not to overuse an inflamed joint, and don't do any exercise that causes any pain or discomfort.

Question 10   If your knee hurts when you walk down steps, it's a sign of weakness in your knee joint. You may have injured your knee at some point in your life, or the muscles supporting your knee, your quads and hamstrings, may be weak and/or inflexible. So please follow my advice for people with problem knee joints later in this chapter.

Question 11   If you suffer from headaches, it is often a sign of weakness in the neck and shoulder joints. To avoid further aggravating your problem, please follow my advice for people with neck and shoulder issues. Watch your posture! Poor posture is a major cause of neck and shoulder pain.

Question 12   I have found that people who spend a great deal of time working at a computer are prone to neck and shoulder problems, even if they don't realize it. Take a break from the screen every 20 minutes and be sure to do your shoulder and neck stretches.

Question 13   If you have pain or discomfort in your shoulders or neck when you lift things over your head, it's a sign of a weakness in the upper body area. You should work on improving your shoulder strength and flexibility.

Question 14   When I ask clients if they are flexible, they'll often answer, "Yes, but I can't straighten my leg," or "Sure, but I can't touch my toes," or "I have trouble lifting my arms over my head." This question is designed to make you aware of any tightness that you may have in your body that may need special attention.

Question 15   If you are popping over-the-counter or prescription pain medication to relieve aching joints or sore muscles, it's likely that you have arthritis or another type of joint problem. Please get to the real cause of your pain or discomfort so that you can best treat it. Are you taking medication because you get headaches, which may be caused by tightness or weakness in your neck and shoulders? Are you trying to relieve the pain of an aching back or pain in the hip socket? Once you identify the cause of your pain you can begin to take the appropriate steps to deal with it without resorting to medication.

Question 16   In my experience, people who routinely visit chiropractors usually go to them because they have back problems. If you are regularly seeing a chiropractor, your back probably feels better for it, but you still have an underlying problem that needs watching. So follow my workout advice for people with weak or painful backs.

strengthening your weak links

If you found that you have one or two or even more weak links, don't feel bad. No body is perfect, and I mean that literally. Just about everyone has a weak area somewhere on his or her body that needs extra attention. It could be an aching back or a creaky knee—or maybe it's a real pain in the neck. Wherever it may be, ignore your weak link(s) at your own peril. If you don't strengthen your weak links, they will get weaker. Over time, weak links may interfere with your ability to maintain an active lifestyle. When people are in pain, they tend to shy away from working out or even just taking a walk. Pain breeds inactivity; inactivity breeds more pain and more injury. The solution is to pay attention to your weak links before they cause lasting damage.

Although exercise is wonderful for strengthening muscles and improving joint flexibility, people with particular problems need to avoid

Treating an Acute Injury the RICE Way

RICE is an acronym for rest, ice, compression, elevation.

RICE is the treatment of choice for the first forty-eight hours following an immediate injury to a soft tissue such as a pulled tendon or muscle strain.

Rest   If you are in pain, don't work out or overexert yourself. Give yourself time to heal. Sit down or lie down and stay off the injury!

Ice   Apply an ice pack to the injured area for 10 to 15 minutes at a time every hour or so. You can put some ice in a plastic zip bag, or you can even use a package of frozen peas (in the plastic bag). Or you can do as I do—fill a bunch of paper cups halfway with water and put them in the freezer. Then, when you need to ice an injury or sore muscle, just grab one of the cups, peel off the paper down to the ice, and then do a slow ice massage on the injury for about five minutes. This really helps to reduce pain and inflammation.

Compression   Wrap an elastic bandage (such as an ACE bandage) around the injury. This helps reduce swelling and relieves inflammation. Make sure the bandage is wrapped firmly but not so tightly that you cut off circulation to the area.

Elevation   While you are resting, place a pillow under the injured area and keep it slightly elevated. If you can sleep in this position, all the better.

exercises that may aggravate their condition. This doesn't mean that you shouldn't exercise your weak links, but it does mean that you need to be careful about how you do it.

your aching back

About 80 percent of all North Americans suffer from at least one backache in their lifetime, and for many, lower back pain is a chronic condition. Fortunately, in most cases, lower back pain can be successfully treated with the right combination of strength training, sensible stretching, and improved posture. Regular workouts will reduce pain by strengthening the muscles that support your back and by improving your flexibility.

A sedentary lifestyle is bad for your back. Don't sit in one position for too long. Get up and stretch your legs every few minutes; this will take pressure off your back and keep your blood flowing. If possible, avoid long car trips. If you have to sit in a car or an airplane for a long period of time, take frequent breaks to get up and walk around. Be sure to maintain excellent posture. Do your posture check often! An imbalance in your back muscles will make your back vulnerable to injury. In addition, be sure that your mattress is firm enough to support your back and that your pillows are in proper alignment on your bed. Don't sleep on your stomach; this will weaken your back muscles. Sleep on your side, with your knees tucked in a fetal position. And be sure that your desk chair provides proper support for your lower back. If your lower back is not flush against the back of the seat, you can use a small pillow for support at the base of your spine.

As much as I am an advocate of stretching, I urge people with back problems to be very careful when they stretch. When the back is tight, the back muscles and joints are not able to achieve a full range of motion. If you push a muscle too far, it could go into spasm and cause further injury. If you do stretch, do so gently and carefully and don't push. Avoid any exercises or stretches that involve rotating your back and/or twisting your spine, such as the Oblique Crunch. Rotating your spine could easily throw your back out of alignment and cause pain. The Hamstring Stretch, the Knee-Chest Stretch, and the Side Back Stretch are good stretches for your back if you can do them without pain.

Hamstring Stretch

The hamstring stretch improves flexibility in the back of the thigh, which takes pressure off your lower back.

1. Sit on the floor with one leg stretched out and the other leg folded in, with the bottom of your foot resting inside the knee of your extended leg.

2. Lean forward, pointing your fingertips toward your toes. Do

not bend over. Keep your spine straight. Do not tug, pull, or yank—just gently point toward your toes.

3. Feel a relaxed stretch in the back of the thigh of your extended leg. Hold for 20 seconds. Repeat two times, then switch legs and do the other side.

Knee-Chest Stretch

This simple stretch is great at relieving nagging lower back pain. It improves back muscle flexibility, and is a *must* for anyone who has chronic back pain.

1. Lie flat on your back. Gently pull both knees in toward your chest until you feel a mild stretch in your lower back. This should feel good, not painful. If you like, you can wrap a towel around your feet and hold it with your hands to help with the stretch.

2. Hold the stretch for 30 seconds. Don't bounce or pull, just hold the position.

3. Release the stretch. Rest 30 seconds and repeat two times.

Side Back Stretch

Don't do this exercise when you're in pain. Do it when you feel better and want to strengthen your core muscles so that they better support your back. Keep it up and maybe you'll be out of pain forever.

1. Get on all fours on the floor. Tuck in your stomach muscles and keep your lower back in a neutral position. Don't let your back sag down or arch up.

2. Extend your right leg and your left arm simultaneously to around shoulder level. Hold for 15 seconds. Return to the starting position.

3. Repeat the exercise with your left leg and right arm. Do 6 to 10 repetitions on both sides.

If you have back problems, never exercise cold back muscles. Normally, I consider the first set of any exercise to be the warm-up set, but that may not be enough of a warm-up for people with chronic back pain. If you have chronic back pain, I recommend that you do 5 to 10 minutes of back-friendly aerobic exercise to warm up your muscles before working out. Running, jogging, and jumping rope should be avoided because they are rough on your back and joints (not to mention your knees). The repetitive motion of the treadmill can also aggravate back pain. If you have access to a pool, swimming is great because you work all the muscles in your back without stressing your body. If you use an exercise bicycle at home or at the gym, be sure to use a recumbent bike, which offers back support, not the standard bike, which causes too much compression on the spine. Power walking is fine as long as you maintain the proper posture and it doesn't hurt your back. Walking actually puts less strain on the spine than unsupported sitting, and only slightly more than standing. Be sure to wear good walking shoes that give you good support. If any form of aerobic exercise hurts your back, you can always warm up with a heating pad. Lie with your back flat on the floor on a warm, moist heating pad covered with a towel for about 10 minutes. This helps to bring blood to your back muscles, warming them up for the workout.

Some exercises are not appropriate for people with back problems. If you have chronic back pain, avoid lifting extremely heavy weights. Try to work within a moderate Level 3 of intensity on the Noble Rating Scale. Do not do squats with a barbell or use a leg press with a heavy setting, because these exercises put too much pressure on your spine. Use your common sense. If you begin to get into position to an exercise and it feels as if it's putting too much pressure on your back, stop! Don't push yourself. Try it again another day and see if it feels better.

acute back pain

You reach down to tie your shoe or you move the wrong way and you throw your back out. Suddenly, you're in a great deal of pain. Don't try to exercise or stretch on your own. For the first forty-eight hours after the initial incident, rest is best. Get off your feet and try to find a comfortable position. Put an ice pack on the affected area and repeat every ten minutes for as long as needed. A warm shower or a moist heating pad can sometimes bring relief. An over-the-counter nonsteroidal anti-inflammatory medication such as ibuprofen or aspirin every four hours can help reduce inflammation and pain. These medications should be used only for a short time. If pain persists, you should see your doctor.

The real solution is to get to the root cause of the pain. It could be due to a general weakness in the muscles supporting the back. Many people with back pain have disk alignment problems. If a displaced disk presses on a spinal nerve, it can send shooting pain down the hip and back, causing a condition called sciatica. If you are in a great deal of pain, call your doctor. He or she will probably give you the same advice that I did, but in rare cases, he or she may want to see you for further examination. After the acute episode passes, ask your doctor whether you should get a course of physical therapy with a trained rehabilitation therapist who can show you exercises to strengthen your back and improve your flexibility safely. In many cases, physical therapy may be covered by your medical insurance. You should also consider seeking the help of a chiropractor, a practitioner who treats injuries and illness through adjustment and manipulation of the spinal column. In my experience, chiropractors are great at treating lower back pain and preventing future back problems. They are experts at keeping your spinal vertebrae in alignment, which can help prevent disk problems and other imbalances that can cause pain and injury.

weak in the knees

Knee injuries are also extremely common; they are the number-one reason people visit orthopedic surgeons. The knee joint is formed by the junction of the tibia, or shinbone; the femur, or thighbone; and the patella, or kneecap. Although the knee is built to withstand a tremendous amount of pressure, we often overtax it. A sharp or sudden twisting motion can tear a ligament supporting the knee joint. A blow to the kneecap can cause a wearing down of the cartilage, the protective covering on bones that keeps them from rubbing against each other. Excessive running or time on a stair machine can wear knee joints down. If you want problem-free knees, it is extremely important to keep the supporting muscles (quadricep muscles) surrounding the knee joint strong so that the knee joint doesn't have to pick up the slack. If you engage in a sport involving running, jumping, or pivoting, be sure to wear the right shoes for your sport—preferably ones that are well cushioned—so that the impact from the ground is absorbed by the shoe and not the knee.

Knee injuries are very common among skiers. Skiers—especially weekend warriors—must be careful about maintaining their leg muscles all year long so that they don't blow their knees out their first day on the slopes. If you are not following a serious strength-training program, be cautious about getting on skis.

If you have any knee problems, don't do knee bends. When you exercise, be very careful about the position of your knees in relation to your toes. Your knees should never extend over your toes; rather, they should be aligned straight under your hips. Do not lock your knees, and don't yank at them when you stretch. Be gentle!

Here's a great exercise to help strengthen the quadricep muscle that supports the knee.

For Strong Quads

1. Sit on an exercise ball with both feet flat on the ground. Hold your stomach in and focus on keeping your core stable.

2. Slowly extend your right leg while contracting your quads. Squeeze the muscle in as you gently lift your leg. Do not fully extend your knee, as this will cause more pain.

3. Hold for 2 seconds and release. Do 10 repetitions, and then repeat the exercise on your left leg.

a pain in the neck

If you sit in front of a computer screen all day long holding your head in one position, or if you spend hours a day chatting with the phone nestled between your shoulder and your ear, you probably have experienced neck pain. In most cases, neck pain is caused by poor posture resulting from sitting, working, or sleeping in an awkward position. Stress is another major culprit. Many people carry the weight of the world on their neck and shoulders. The minute they feel under pressure, they tighten up their muscles in the upper back and neck. Over time, the muscles get sore and tired. In most cases, there is a simple solution for chronic neck pain. First, make sure that your workspace is well designed so that you don't have to contort your body in a way that harms your neck. Second, try to keep the muscles in your neck and shoulders strong, flexible, and relaxed.

Working out is a great way to strengthen your muscles and relieve tension. People with neck problems should not lift heavy objects above their head, as this will only irritate their neck. Be gentle with your stretching. Yanking or jerking your neck can cause injury and pain. Don't sit in one position for too long, especially if you are typing on a keyboard. Get up, walk around, do a few shoulder rolls. Lift your shoulders up to your ears, hold for a few seconds, and release them. Gently roll your head from side to side. Take a few deep breaths and relax.

Here's a neck exercise you can do right at your desk.

Desk Chair Neck Relaxer

1. Sit up straight in your chair with your feet on the floor in front of you. Reach down and grasp the underside of the seat or its rear leg with your right hand.
2. Turn your head all the way to the left, then look down. With your left hand, gently grasp the top back of your head. Don't pull; just hold firmly enough to maintain the left-look-down position.

3. Lean forward toward your left side and feel a mild stretch in your right neck area from the top of the shoulder blade to the base of the neck. Hold this position and visualize the muscles relaxing.

4. Repeat and hold the stretch on the left side for 30 to 60 seconds. Exhale as you feel your muscles relax. Gently release.

5. Repeat on your right side to stretch-out your left neck area. Do this stretch several times throughout the day as you take your regular breaks from sitting, phone, and keyboard work.

don't neglect your shoulders

The shoulder muscles are particularly vulnerable to injury, primarily because we tend to abuse them. Most people do not properly strengthen the entire shoulder area but rather concentrate on one or two muscle groups and forget about the rest. Moreover, poor posture (sitting or standing in a slouched position with your shoulders hunched forward) can gradually weaken your shoulder muscles. To add insult to injury, few people properly stretch their shoulder muscles after working out, which leaves them tight and inflexible. This creates imbalances in the shoulder region, which will inevitably lead to injury. If you don't have any shoulder problems, I urge you to follow the entire Body Noble Program so that you build strong, flexible shoulder muscles.

Here's what can happen if you don't. One day, you might reach for a suitcase in the overhead compartment of a train or airplane, and your shoulder will go into spasm. This common injury is known as a rotator cuff injury and it can be quite painful, but if you take proper care of your shoulders, it doesn't have to happen to you.

If you have a shoulder problem, please check with your physician or physiotherapist before doing any exercises.

If you have acute shoulder problems, don't lift anything heavy over your head, and don't do the overhead press exercise at the gym or with weights. It is critical for you to keep your rotator cuff muscles strong and flexible. Here's a great exercise for your rotator cuff.

Rotator Cuff Exercise

1. Tie one end of your exercise cable to a doorknob or a stair banister and hold the free end in your right hand. Facing the door or banister, bend your right arm 90 degrees, keeping your right elbow close at your side.

2. Pull the cable away from your body and then release it back in toward you. Repeat the exercise. Do two sets of 15 repetitions. Switch arms and repeat the exercise on the other arm. Do the Rotator Cuff Stretch after this exercise.

> **Noble Tip**
>
> While doing this exercise, imagine that your working elbow is a door hinge that is opening and closing as you pull the cable in and out.

Rotator Cuff Stretch

1. Keep your right arm bent 90 degrees while keeping your right elbow close to your side, similar to the starting position for the Rotator Cuff Exercise.

2. Place your right hand on the edge of the wall while still keeping your elbow at your side. Slightly turn your body away from the wall until you feel the stretch in your upper shoulder. Hold the stretch for 15 seconds, and then repeat the stretch on the other arm.

healthy hips

Hip injuries are not as common as back, knee, or shoulder injuries, but they can cause a great deal of discomfort for the unfortunate few who have them. Keeping your hip muscles strong and hip joints flexible can prevent most hip problems. It's also important to keep the muscles surrounding your hips flexible, including the gluteal muscles, hip flexors, hamstrings, and quadriceps. If you have pain in your hip area, avoid doing lunges or squatting exercises. These movements will put too great a strain on your hip muscles and joints.

Although not directly related to the hip muscles, sciatica (the impingement of the sciatica nerve by a disk in the spine) can cause pain in the hip region. Typically, sciatica causes shooting pain from the lower back down through the thigh. If you have sciatica, do not do any exercises that involve the buttocks or gluteal muscles while you are in pain because they can further irritate the area.

The best exercise to strengthen hip muscles is the band hip extension, as described below.

Exercise Cable Side Leg Raise

See photos and directions on page 89.

it's all in the wrist

There have been numerous fitness books devoted to improving your abs, tightening your thighs, and sculpting your butt, but not a single one about strengthening your wrists! I know there is no cosmetic payoff to exercising your wrist joints, but keeping your wrist flexors strong could pay off in other ways—it could help keep you gainfully employed. If you spend a great deal of time typing on a keyboard, punching a cash register, cutting hair, performing surgery, or doing any job that requires the repeated flexing or tensing of your wrist, hand, or fingers, you are at risk of developing carpal tunnel syndrome. Symptoms of carpal tunnel syndrome include shooting pains down your arms, wrist pain, and/or numbness in your hands and fingers. If you have any of these symptoms, you should see a doctor specializing in repetitive stress injuries. Early intervention can make a real difference by nipping a small problem in the bud. In most cases, carpal tunnel syndrome is treated with an exercise rehabilitation program. In severe cases, surgery may be required or even a change of occupation. Prevention is the best approach. If you want to avoid the problem in the first place, it is critical to strengthen the muscles supporting your wrists and to keep them flexible. Creating a work station that is well designed for your body can help prevent carpal tunnel syndrome and other repetitive stress injuries. Here is an easy exercise designed to strengthen your wrist extensors.

Wrist Strengthener

1. Grab a light dumbbell (2 to 5 pounds) in one hand, palm down, with the arm parallel to the floor and supported on your thigh or a table.
2. Let the weight of the dumbbell bend your wrist forward or down, and then draw your knuckles upward toward the ceiling. You will feel the work in your forearm muscles and wrist.
3. Repeat the exercise 15 to 20 times on both hands.

Wrist Stretch

1. Face a table, or any other horizontal surface that is about mid-thigh level. Step forward with one leg, placing your foot beneath the table.
2. Lean forward over the table and position your hands—palms down, fingers straight out and pointing back toward you—flat onto the table. Gently lean back so that you feel a mild stretch on the underside of your forearms.
3. Try to grip the table with both hands, as if you were palming a basketball. Hold the stretch for 30 to 60 seconds. Repeat the exercise with your palms facing up.

noble looks

You're taking care of your body by working out, eating well, and taking your supplements. You deserve to look your best from head to toe. Here are some ways you can pamper yourself so that you look as good as you feel.

skin deep

I was trained as a body treatment specialist at one of the most highly respected spas in the world, La Prairie Spa, located at the Beverly Hills Hotel. Our clientele included Hollywood celebrities with seemingly bottomless pocketbooks. One of the most popular treatments was the diamond deluxe body scrub. That's right, diamonds! Finely ground diamonds are made into a body scrub to exfoliate dead skin cells, leaving the skin smooth and glowing. This was the most expensive treatment offered at the spa.

Trust me, you don't have to break the bank to have good skin. There are lots of things you can do that are relatively inexpensive but that work as well. Skin is not just a cosmetic covering, it's the largest organ system in the body. Skin performs many vital tasks in the body, including providing a barrier against bacteria, viruses, fungi, and other toxins that can do us harm. Skin is essential for maintaining your body temperature. Skin enables us to retain blood and water, which are essential for life. Skin is also key to the production and absorption of vitamin D, which is essential for the absorption of calcium in the body. Taking care of your skin is not a matter of vanity, it is essential for good health.

When I talk about skin care, I'm not talking about just the stuff you put on the outside of your body; skin care begins on the inside. Someone who is eating a nutrient-poor diet, especially a diet that does not contain enough good oils, is going to have dry, lifeless skin, hair, and nails. The first step to achieving great skin is to follow my Noble Nutrition plan and to be sure to take your essential fatty oils every day. In Noble Nutrition, I recommend taking 1 tablespoon of good oil daily either in your protein shake or on your salad. Do it!

When you work out, you dehydrate your body, and that includes your skin, so rehydrate yourself from the inside out and the outside in. If you don't drink enough water, your skin will dry out. Please drink 8 cups of purified water daily. If you find water boring, liven it up with a twist of lemon, lime, or orange or a splash of fresh juice.

Getting enough sleep is also important for good skin. There is no effective remedy for those annoying dark shadows under your eyes that are caused by lack of sleep. You can use coverups to lighten them a bit, but the fact is, a good night's sleep is the best way to get rid of them. Your body is busy working away while you're sleeping—while you're off dreaming, your body is secreting human growth hormone and other skin growth factors that stimulate the production of new skin cells. So try to get 7 to 8 hours of sleep on most nights.

If you want to keep your skin wrinkle-free, don't smoke and don't expose your skin to secondhand smoke. The toxins in smoke create free radicals in your skin that can promote the formation of wrinkles. Did you know that smokers' skin looks at least five years older than the skin of nonsmokers? You may not care about that at age twenty, but believe me, by age thirty-five you're not going to want to look forty or older.

I am a strong advocate of using only natural products devoid of harsh chemicals. Don't use standard soap on your face or body, because it is too drying. Avoid anything with alcohol, which can also dry out your skin. Even if you have oily skin, you need to maintain some moisture. Wash your face with a natural facial cleanser that does not contain alcohol or other ingredients that strip skin of its natural oils. Use a nonabrasive body wash or Pears soap (a glycerin-based soap) in the bath or shower. I also love Aveda products, but Neutrogena and Oil of Olay make excellent skin care products that you can find in any drugstore. I recommend buying products designed for sensitive skin that don't contain irritants such as dyes or fragrances. Use a bath shower glove or a body net bath sponge to exfoliate dead skin. Be sure that the shower glove and sponge are not too caustic against your skin. Keep a pumice stone on hand in the shower to treat calluses or rough spots on your feet.

If you have dry skin, apply a body moisturizer after you shower. Some good brands include Lubriderm, Keri Lotion, Kiehls, and Neutrogena, which are available at most pharmacies and discount stores. I recommend using unscented lotions because they are less irritating and don't clash with the fragrance of your favorite perfume or aftershave.

Be sure to cleanse your face after you work out to get rid of the sweat and dirt. The Noble Rule for skin care is not to do anything to irritate your skin. Respect it. Treat it kindly. First, rinse your face with warm, not hot, water. Second, apply your facial cleanser to your face. Massage gently. Don't scrub the cleanser off with a washcloth. Splash warm water on your face to gently rinse it off, and then pat your face dry lightly. Apply a toner that is suited for your skin type—normal, normal oily, normal dry, sensitive, problem (adult acne), or combination. Then apply a light, non-oil-based moisturizer on your face to keep your skin soft and prevent dryness.

Many women and men today use special skin care products, cosmeceuticals, that are designed to prevent or even erase age-related lines and wrinkles. Cosmeceuticals include antioxidant vitamins and herbs that are applied directly to the skin to prevent wear and tear. Some skin care products sold in fancy department stores can run you into the hundreds of dollars, but the most expensive ones are not necessarily the best. What goes in the jar is more important than fancy packaging or advertising. I have found some of the brands sold in health food stores to be excellent and well priced. A good vitamin C is one of the best things you can put on your skin, but it has to be in the right form or it won't get absorbed. Vitamin C appears to stimulate the formation of new collagen, which helps keep skin from sagging, and it fills in wrinkle lines, giving your skin a fresh, healthy look. There are some excellent vitamin C creams in all price ranges, ranging from about $100 a jar to under $15. Cellex C and Skinceuticals are among the pricier brands, but they give excellent results. Ester C produced by DermaE is more for the budget conscious, but is also a fine product.

For best results, I like to combine antioxidant creams. In addition to vitamin C, I recommend using creams containing alpha lipoic acid, co-enzyme Q10, vitamin E, and green tea extract, all powerful antioxidants. The phytochemicals pycnogenol (an extract from pine tree bark) and astazanthin (an extract from plant algae) included in some better skin care products will also give your skin a healthy glow. Don't use any products near your eyes unless they are specifically for under-eye care. The skin under your eyes is very sensitive and needs special care.

Moisturizers containing hyaluronic acid are especially good for people with dry skin. Hyaluronic acid binds moisture to skin cells and helps keep skin smoother and more elastic.

Every week or so, I recommend using a natural nonabrasive scrub on your face to get rid of the dead cells. This leaves the skin looking brighter and fresher. There are several good ones on the market, including Aveda, Neutrogena, St. Ives, and Clinique. A nonabrasive scrub feels smooth and creamy, and isn't harsh.

Treat yourself to a professional facial on a regular basis if you can afford it. Women should try to get a facial every month or so, and men around four times a year. A facial cleanses your skin right down to the pores and rids your face of dead cells. It's also a very pleasant, relaxing experience.

A specially trained esthetician performs the facial. A typical facial begins with a gentle cleansing of the skin and neck. This is followed by a few minutes of steam directed at the face to open up the pores, which are often clogged with oil and dirt. After the steam treatment, an exfoliant is massaged into the skin to remove dead cells. The exfoliation may be followed by a process called a skin extraction in which the pores are cleaned using a metal extractor. This has to be done very gently or else it can hurt. After the extraction, a skin mask usually containing herbs and vitamins may be placed on the face for a few minutes to nourish the skin. After the mask is removed, a light moisturizer is applied to the skin, and you're good to go.

the at-home noble facial routine

If you just can't fit a professional facial into your budget, you can give yourself an at-home facial for a fraction of the price and get reasonably good results. You'll have to invest in a few skin care products, but it's still going to cost a lot less than a salon facial.

Before you begin, organize your skin care products as listed below.

1. A gentle facial cleanser
2. A prepackaged mixture of your favorite dried herbs (whatever smells good is fine!)
3. A gentle exfoliant
4. A skin mask
5. A moisturizer

Cleanse   Start your at-home facial by gently cleansing your skin with your regular cleanser. Pat your skin dry.

Steam   Boil 2 quarts of water. Add 2 tablespoons of your favorite dried herbs. Carefully remove the pot from the heat and put it on a heat-resistant surface on a table. Sit about 1 foot away from the pot.

Using a towel, make a tentlike cover over your head as you lean over the hot pot. Take a few deep relaxing breaths. Let the steam seep into your skin, getting deep into your pores. Steam your face for about 5 minutes.

Exfoliant　Gently massage the nonabrasive exfoliant into your skin. Rinse it off.

Skin Mask　Carefully apply your favorite skin mask to your face, avoiding your eyes. Remove the mask in 10 minutes with a warm washcloth.

Moisturizer　Gently apply your moisturizer.

Look at yourself in the mirror. Your skin should look brighter, smoother, and healthier.

Whenever you go outdoors, be sure to wear the right sunscreen on your face and exposed portions of your body. There are two types of ultraviolet rays: UVA and UVB. Both stimulate the formation of free radicals in the skin, which promote wrinkles and other signs of aging and cancer. These are the same free radicals that promote aging inside the body. Your sunscreen should protect against both types of rays. Ombrelle makes a terrific broad-spectrum sunblock lotion. It is waterproof and completely non-oily, and it goes on easily and doesn't feel sticky. If you like to look tan, I recommend using a natural cosmetic bronzer on your face. Nearly every major cosmetic company has a bronzer on the market, and they work fine as long as you follow the directions. (If you don't apply your bronzer with care, you can leave dark streaks on your skin.)

hair care

A great hairstyle can complement all the hard work you are doing for your body to look great. Having been on television for so many years, I have worked with a lot of hairstylists, and they all agree that the most important thing you can do for your hair is to get the right cut. No product can compensate for a hairstyle that is not suited to your face. How do you find a great stylist? Ask friends for referrals or check out local magazines for articles about salons in your area. Interview the stylist before you allow him or her to put scissors to your hair. Bring in pictures of hairstyles from magazines that you think would look good on you. Once you get the right style, maintain it by getting a trim every month or so.

If you work out a lot, sweat a great deal, or live in a city with dirty air, you're going to need to wash your hair every day. Avoid shampoos and conditioners with harsh cleansers or chemicals. Don't use the same shampoo every day, because even the best shampoo can leave some buildup. Switch brands every few shampoos, and you will see a real difference in terms of body and shine. I like several brands of hair care products, including Aveda and Neutrogena, which are sold in most pharmacies and discount drugstores, and Bioelements, which is sold in department stores.

body hair

Clients often ask me questions about the best way to remove body hair. My reply is to do what's most comfortable for you. Women can either wax or shave their legs. Although waxing is not painless, it does remove hair at a deeper level and slows down hair growth. Most women use plain old-fashioned razors and not electric razors, because the electric ones often leave stubble. If you choose to shave, be sure to use a shaving cream designed for sensitive skin that prevents nicks and shaving bumps. Aveeno makes an excellent shaving cream for sensitive skin, which incidentally can also be used by men.

Men with sensitive skin should avoid using aftershave lotions that contain alcohol or other chemicals. I use Aveda shaving products, but there are other excellent brands on the market, including Neutrogena and Nivea.

I don't recommend waxing for men to remove body hair. If men have excess hair on their legs, I recommend using electric clippers at a low setting. This will remove your hair without tearing up your skin. If your hair grows in quickly, you will need to remove the stubble more frequently to keep your skin smooth.

If you want to try a depilatory to remove body hair, Nair and Veet are good brands, but they are not for everybody. I don't recommend these products for sensitive skin because many people find them to be irritating. Do a skin test prior to using the product to make sure that you are not allergic to it.

your fitness wardrobe

When you feel good about how you look, you tend to perform better, which is why I recommend that people work out in clothes that flatter their bodies and make them feel attractive. Treat yourself to some hip, sexy, functional clothes that will make you want to work out. There are numerous lines of fitness clothing on the market in all price ranges. I have designed a functional line of clothes for FitTV that are stylized for the active person on the go. I chose a light cotton line because the fabric feels soft and comfortable next to the body and prevents the body from overheating. Workout clothes should fit well and not be too tight or confining. I'm not against all synthetic fabrics; unlike the old polyesters that held in heat and moisture, some of the newer, high-tech fabrics are designed to let your body breathe. Be sure to buy fabrics that wick moisture away from your body so that you stay cool and comfortable. I recommend that you go to a quality sporting goods store and check out the clothing lines, or explore the Internet. You will be amazed at the amount of great fitness clothing to choose from for every taste and pocketbook.

It's important to dress correctly for the season and the activity. If you're out power walking in the hot summer, wear as little as possible to keep cool. Be sure to use sunscreen, and wear a visor if the sun bothers you. (A hat may be too warm.) Your water bottle is your most important fashion accessory—don't leave home without it.

If you're doing outdoor activity in cooler weather, be sure to dress in layers so that if you warm up, you can take off your jacket or sweater and tie it around your waist.

If you work out indoors at your office or a gym, always keep a light pair of long pants and a light coverup handy, because some indoor spaces are very over-air-conditioned, and you don't want to get a muscle cramp from the cold. As you warm up during your workout, you can strip down to your shorts and T-shirt.

Here are some clothing items that I recommend you keep in your closet as part of your fitness wardrobe. You may want to choose a high-performance version designed to whisk away sweat and to keep you dry during your workout.

Lightweight tops, one long-sleeve, one short-sleeve

Tank tops and workout shorts

Workout jackets or long-sleeve fleece tops

Long pants with a drawstring or elastic waist

Cotton and high-performance socks

An outdoor nylon shell top and pants for cold-weather outdoor activities

Running shoes

Cross-training shoes

A lifestyle shoe for your sport or activity

2 fitted sports bras for women

the right footwear

Wearing the right footwear is essential to preventing injury. I recommend that you purchase your footwear at a reputable sporting goods store or athletic footwear store where you can have a knowledgeable salesperson help you make your selection.

Match the shoe to your activity. Running shoes have more padding in the front and on the balls of the feet than walking shoes or tennis shoes and are designed for people running in a straight line. Tennis shoes have more side padding because unlike runners, tennis players are more likely to move from side to side to hit the ball. Walking shoes have slightly different foot boxes than running, tennis, or cross-training shoes. Cross-training shoes are more lightweight than traditional running shoes and can be used for tennis or short running sessions but not long-distance running. Shoe manufacturers have invested a lot of time and money in designing shoes with different technical requirements. Take advantage of their hard work. My favorite brand is New Balance, but for fashion I love my Pumas and Nikes.

Buy a shoe that fits your foot. Don't assume you know your shoe size. Be sure to have your foot measured every time you buy shoes, because your feet can keep growing in adulthood. It's not unusual to gain a full shoe size during adulthood. Remember that all feet are not the same shape—you need to find a shoe that is suited to your type of foot. Some of the better footwear manufacturers offer shoes in a variety of widths, from narrow to wide. If your foot is not a standard medium width, don't be talked into buying a shoe that is not your correct size. You will never be comfortable in it, and it could cause instability in your gait, which can result in injury. The best time to shop for shoes is late afternoon, when your feet are more swollen than they are earlier in the day. Try your shoes on with the same pair of socks that you will wear when you are working out or doing your sport.

Buy two pairs of athletic shoes so that you don't wear the same pair every day. Plan on replacing your shoes every year—even if you don't wear them down, the rubber becomes rigid.

Open-back athletic shoes (slides), the latest rage, are fine to wear running errands or walking around town, but they are not stable enough for serious walking or other activities. They are for fashion, not fitness.

your body noble in-home day spa

If you have the time and money, there is no better way to unwind than to spend the day at a spa. But there are ways you can indulge your need to pamper yourself right in your home that are much cheaper. I have developed a great at-home routine for my clients that leaves them feeling relaxed and refreshed.

Epsom Salts Bath   Buy a bag of Epsom salts at your local pharmacy or discount drugstore. Fill your tub with comfortably hot water. Add around 3 cups of salt. Light your favorite scented candle and put on a soothing CD. Soak in the tub for about 20 minutes. Treat yourself to an Epsom salt bath once a week. It's a great way to unwind, and it helps prevent muscle soreness after your workout. (Women should not do this treatment during menstruation.) If you use Epsom salts, drink a lot of water.

Cold Water Effusion   This is my favorite treatment to soothe my legs after a long run or hard leg workout. After you have completed your shower, step back from the shower and turn on the cold water for 1 minute. First, put your right leg in the stream of water and rotate the leg so that the water first moves down the front then your glutes and the back of your legs. Then switch to the other leg. This treatment helps you get rid of some of the lactic acid that may have accumulated after your run or workout. It also speeds up recovery.

Tennis Ball Massage   This is a great way to get rid of knots in your back muscles. Stand near a flat, unobstructed wall. Hold a tennis ball on the area of your back that is feeling stiff and sore. Push your back and ball gently into the wall and hold it in this position for 30 seconds. Focus on exhaling as you squeeze your back into the ball. Feel your muscles begin to relax from the pressure of the ball.

Ball Foot Reflexology   Reflexology is a therapy that works on the feet to promote the healing of the entire body. Reflexologists believe that pressure points in the feet correlate to different parts of your body and that by relieving stress in the feet, you can promote overall wellness. Many spas offer reflexology foot massage treatments. Here's a simple treatment you can do by yourself. Place a tennis ball on the floor and put your foot on the ball. Rotate your foot over the ball for 1 minute. Switch to the other foot. This treatment will alleviate some of the tension in your feet and help reinvigorate your entire body.

Treating yourself and your body with care is another way to stay connected to yourself. It's worth the investment in yourself. You will feel healthier and happier and will be more likely to continue your fitness program.

16

the noble spirit: finding your balance

The phrase "body, mind, and spirit," has become so overused these days that it is in danger of becoming a meaningless slogan. That would be a real shame. The underlying message of the interconnection between the physical, the mental, and the spiritual is an important one. I have my own personal philosophy on this often used expression.

I believe that we need to examine all of the different dimensions of life to live a truly complete life. Too often, we overemphasize one aspect of life over another and we shortchange ourselves in the process. Working in Hollywood, I meet many people who are solely concerned about their physical selves, who work out for hours a day and are preoccupied with their diets, clothes, and exterior appearances. I also meet my share of spiritual junkies who spend their days meditating, praying, or seeking spiritual enlightenment and who neglect their brains and their bodies. The vast majority of people I meet are what I call mind-focused, completely engulfed in professional pursuits, while neglecting other vital components of life. Given the amount of time most of us spend in school and on the job, it's easy to become mind-focused and we are often rewarded for it—at least at first. But in the long run, neglecting your body will affect your quality of life. Ultimately, it will destroy your spirit. I know that most educated people intellectually understand the need to take care of their bodies but are somehow stuck in their limited view of life. Instead of trying to figure out how to incorporate fitness in their lives, they look for excuses as to why they don't have time.

The real reason people don't take care of their bodies has very little to do with time. Who can't fit in 20 minutes 3 times a week? The real problem confronting many mind-focused people is an inborn resistance to connecting with their bodies in a positive way. The real question is, why?

Is your resistance rooted in a past experience? Being the school klutz can scar you for life unless you free yourself of that stereotype. Are you too hard on yourself, constantly comparing yourself to supermodels or actresses? Do you believe that you can't ever achieve fitness, so why bother? A huge myth! Everyone can be fit. Do you feel that taking care of yourself is a luxury and that you can't afford the time?

Whatever your reason, you need to accept the fact that something is holding you back. Self-awareness is the first step to becoming unstuck. On days when you can't summon up the energy to work out, or you find yourself looking for excuses not to pursue your fitness program, think about why you may be so reluctant to stay on the program. It probably has more to do with your past than your current situation.

There are simple steps you can take to help reduce the resistance and make you feel more positive about fitness.

- *You must want to be fit.* You must find a place to put the doubt and I-can't-do-it attitude so that you can move forward.

- *You must decide to do it.* When you really commit to pursuing a fit lifestyle, you will find ways to fit it into your life. The insurmountable excuses no longer seem insurmountable.

- *Be consistent.* The longer you stick with a program, the more likely it is you will make it a permanent part of your life. Find a workout buddy who will push you on days when you don't feel like doing it, and vice versa. Program a reminder on your computer to send you an e-mail every day outlining your workout goals for the day. If you're not computer savvy, write down reminders in your calendar where you list your other important appointments.

Noble Tip

Many people find it helpful to keep a journal in which they can keep track of their fitness program and goals. Write about your feelings before and after you work out. Be honest. Include your negative thoughts as well as your positive accomplishments. This is especially important for people who are resistant to exercise. Your journal will become your best friend. It will spur you on when you feel that you can't keep going.

---

how to stay motivated

Many of you may have had false starts—you began a fitness program with great hope and enthusiasm but within a few weeks or months, you quit. Through the years, I have found that clients who have specific goals are more likely to stick with the program than clients who do not. When I work with clients, I encourage them to establish short-term and long-term goals. A short-term goal should be a simple goal that is attainable within a month's time. For example, you may set the short-term goal of being able to comfortably fit into a pair of slacks that were slightly too tight, or do a mile walk in 12 minutes instead of 15 minutes, or start a Tai Chi class. Your long-term goals can be more ambitious. Do you want to get into great shape so you can enjoy a trip to Europe where you will be walking miles a day? Is there a special event down the road such as a wedding or a school reunion, for which you want to look your best? Do you want to gain endurance so you can participate in a charity bike ride or run for a cause you truly believe in? Do you want to resume doing an activity that you once loved such as skiing, but feel that you aren't in good enough physical shape? Choose the goal that is most likely to inspire you to keep going.

I encourage my clients to make an appointment with a professional photographer every year. It's well worth the money. Dress up for the occasion. Get your hair done and wear a flattering outfit. Most people rarely have professional pictures taken of themselves. It's a great way to keep yourself motivated. If you know that you have to face the camera in six or nine months, you are going to work hard to stay trim and fit and look your best. It's also a great way of keeping track of your progress and letting yourself celebrate how good you can look.

Don't forget to reward yourself for your hard work. Give yourself short-term rewards and long-term rewards. If you are vigilant about doing the Body Noble Workout and are careful about what you eat during the week, treat yourself to your favorite dessert on a weekend or splurge and get yourself a facial or a massage. Buy yourself a special outfit or a designer bathing suit. You've worked hard and you deserve it.

To make it easy for you, I designed the Body Noble Calendar and the Body Noble Journal to help you keep track of your workout schedule and your goals and rewards. You can find both on my Web site at www.bodynoble.com.

Be proud of all the short-term and long-term goals that you've been able to achieve. And continue to strive toward the ones that you have not yet completed. The benefits of the Body Noble Program will not only enhance your day-to-day life—they will last a lifetime.

body noble resource list

www.bodynoble.com

Click onto www.bodynoble.com for your customized online training program. I have designed a supplement program that is geared to your specific body type: lean machine, muscle maker, or fat fighter. The high-quality line is manufactured by Genuine Health and sold in the Body Noble store on the bodynoble.com Web site. The Body Noble store also features in-home fitness equipment, men's skin care products, and fitness lifestyle apparel.

thebodynoble.blogspot.com

Join the online Body Noble community at thebodynoble.blogspot.com. Get encouragement and workout tips from other people following the Body Noble Program.

I recommend the following brands:

Music

www.apple.com/ipod   Enhance your workout by downloading Body Noble audio iFIT workout programs to hip music.

Fitness Products

Lululemon Athletica (stylized fitness apparel)

American Apparel

Gaiam

Footwear

    Saucony

    Asics

    New Balance

    Nike

    Puma

The following is a list of my favorite products that can be found at most health food stores, pharmacies, and natural food markets such as Trader Joe's and Whole Foods.

Skin Care

    Aveda

    Kiehls

    Neutrogena

Protein Powders

    Protein +

    Twinlab

    Met-Rx

    Jarrow

    Nutribiotic (vegan rice protein)

Supplements

    Body Noble Solution Based Supplement Program

    Solaray

    Country Life

    Emer Gen C

Protein Bars

    Organic Food Bar

    Tri-O-Plex

Herbal Teas

Yogi Tea

Traditional Medicinals

Triple Leaf

Meat Substitutes

Morningstar Farms

Gardenburger

Yves Veggie Cuisine

Lightlife Smart Veggie Foods

Eggs

Organic Valley

Eggology (egg whites)

Yogurt

Alta Dena

Brown Cow

Stonyfield Farms

Snacks

Organic Food Bars

Tri-O-Plex

Guiltless Gourmet

Genisoy

Wasa crackers

Sauces and Salad Dressings

Consorzio

Cereals

Quaker Oats

Nature's Path

McCann's Steel Cut Irish Oatmeal

Waffles

Van's All-Natural Gourmet Waffles (wheat free)

Kashi GoLean

Milk Substitutes

Rice Dream

Soy Dream

Silk Soymilk

almond milk

index

ibuprofen, 202, 213
ice cream, 171, 180
immune system, 195
indoor grills, 169
inflammation, 207, 213
injuries
    cycling and, 108
    knee, 213–214
    preexisting, 203, 206
    prevention of, 5, 57
    RICE therapy, 122, 209
    rotator cuff, 216
in-line skating, 117
inner thigh muscles (hip abductors),
    30
    exercises, 90
inositol, 200
insulin, 12, 159, 160, 162, 163
iron, 196
Italian food, 182

jogging, 105–106, 212
joints. *See* bones and joints
journal keeping, 235
juice, 172
jumping jacks, 145
jumping rope, 112–113, 145, 212
junk food, 162

Keri Lotion, 223
Kmart, 55
Knee-Chest Stretch, 210, 211
knees
    arthritic, 108, 203
    rope jumping and, 112
    as weak link, 207, 213–214

lactose intolerance, 170–171
LaLanne, Jack, 12
La Prairie Spa, 221
latisimus muscles (lats), 29, 34, 70–72
L-carnitine, 199–200
lean machines, 9, 15, 18–19, 170
    basic eating plan, 158, 174
    cardio and, 9, 15, 19, 101
    diet tips for, 19
    identification of, 16–18
    intensity level and, 19, 22, 60
    posture concerns, 47
    resistance training, 9, 15, 19, 25
    workout tips for, 19, 22
legs
    blood clots and, 142
    cold water effusion and, 231
    dancing and, 110
    exercises, 59, 83–89, 130–131, 133
    lifting and, 51
    post-cycling stretching, 109
    post-rope jumping stretching, 113
    post-run or -jog stretches, 107
    post-walk stretches, 104
    warm-up stretches, 106
    See also specific muscles
legumes, 160, 162, 165, 178
L-glycine, 200–201
lifting posture, 51–52
L-methionine, 201
Lower-Back Butt Stretch, 59, 94
lower-back muscles (erector spinae), 29
    aching/pain in, 121–122, 206, 207,
        209
    exercises, 59, 93–95, 137
    Touch Training, 35